IRELAND'S HIDDEN MEDICINE

IRELAND'S HIDDEN MEDICINE

An exploration of Irish indigenous medicine from legend and myth to the present day

Rosarie Kingston

AEON

First published in 2021 by
Aeon Books
Hilltop
Lewes BN7 3HS

British Library Cataloguing in Publication Data

A C.I.P. for this book is available from the British Library

ISBN-13: 978-1-91350-497-7

Typeset by Medlar Publishing Solutions Pvt Ltd, India

www.aeonbooks.co.uk

For Julia

CONTENTS

ACKNOWLEDGEMENTS

This book is for any person interested in Irish indigenous medicine. It draws on the work of many scholars, and to these I am deeply indebted. Their work added an extra and valuable dimension to the material recorded by writers such as Lady Gregory and Patrick Logan, as well as the treasure troves that are the National Folklore Collection (NFC) and the writings of Sean Ó Súilleabháin.

The written word may form the warp in the elaboration of thoughts and ideas, but it is conversation that forms the weft, and I have been truly fortunate in this area. Over many years, I have been blessed by the insights of indigenous healers, colleagues, and teachers. These conversations and discussions have expanded and developed my knowledge of traditional medicine in all its guises. My sincere thanks to you all.

Any mistakes and inadequacies in this book are my own, and my apologies if I have not done justice to the many scholars and colleagues who have trodden and illuminated this path for me. Their work is a deeper well from which my readers may drink, if this book whets their appetite to learn more about Irish indigenous medicine.

A special thanks also to Criostóir Mac Carthaig, Director of the National Folklore Collection at University College Dublin, who was so helpful in offering the image of the Pattern day at Glendalough and giving me access to the collection. Thanks also to Clodagh Doyle and Liam Doherty of the National Museum for the images of Brigid crosses.

I thank Kevin for his encyclopaedic knowledge of books and his ability to source a required volume in his vast uncatalogued collection, when the only clue offered was a phrase, or an idea. His knowledge of modern Irish history was of inestimable value, as his collection had many gems I would not have otherwise mined.

Finally, there are my family and friends, whose laughter, wit, kindness, and encouragement, have sustained me for many years now. Thank you all for being your unique selves, as you travel your different walks through life and accompany me on mine. A special thank you Mary and Anita, for the time you spent on proofreading, and your many invaluable comments and insights.

Finally, I thank Aeon Books for publishing this book, thus giving me the opportunity to show the inestimably rich indigenous healing tradition we have in Ireland.

ABOUT THE AUTHOR

Rosarie Kingston practises as a medical herbalist in an integrative medical practice in West Cork, Ireland and lectures on the topic "Herbs and Healing in Irish Folklore" in the Department of Folklore and Ethnology, at University College, Cork.

Like other medical herbalists, her training involved the study of the biological sciences, biomedical diagnostic techniques, and the tradition and science of plants that may be used therapeutically. These seemingly opposite subjects were reconciled in an MSc thesis discussing the scientific foundation for the therapeutic use of *Crataegus monogyna* and a PhD dissertation exploring the rich vein of Irish vernacular medicine in the twenty-first century.

She considers this blending of science and tradition, and the integration of both where possible, to be the best way forward for modern healthcare as it will benefit both the health-care professional and the patient. Her work and involvement with the Irish College of Traditional and Integrative Medicine (ICTIM) in training healthcare professionals to achieve this integration in their practice is, therefore, of paramount importance to her, as it draws together the wisdom and knowledge of different medical traditions with biomedicine.

INTRODUCTION

Ireland's indigenous medicine is a diamond hidden in plain sight. Its beauty is present in our landscape, our festivals, our language, and yet we ignore it to the detriment of our health and wellbeing. The many thousands who climb Croagh Patrick on the last Sunday in July, or the many pilgrims who travel to any one of Ireland's numerous holy wells are aware that such excursions are part of their heritage, but very few see these activities as an integral part of a healing tradition. These journeys are not considered part of medicine, because biomedicine* is the dominant medical system of healthcare in the country and every other means of healing is deemed immaterial, even inconsequential.

The position of biomedicine is not questioned, even though it is a medical system born of a particular time, place, and culture, just as Irish indigenous medicine is. There are other renowned medical systems in the world, such as Ayurveda, Unani, and Chinese medicine, and these too are products of their culture and worldview. In chapter one therefore, I seek to tease out the theories and philosophy that underpin biomedicine to show how they differ, at their very core, to the belief system underlying Irish indigenous medicine. All aspects of

---

*Called biomedicine because it is based on the biological systems of the body.

biomedicine, be it pathology, diagnosis, or therapeutics, are based on the biological systems of a person, resulting in specialists of the cardiovascular system, respiratory system, and endocrine system, among others. The problem affecting a patient's health has to be clearly defined and described, with the subjective symptoms of the patient only relevant in so far as they allow the physician to correlate them to signs that may be seen and measured.

The philosophy of Descartes and Bacon, with their stress on the importance of mathematical certainty, is the foundation on which biomedicine is built and is the opposite to indigenous medicine, where the subjective experience and personal narrative of the patient is deemed all important. Indigenous medicine, no matter where it exists in the world, is characterised by the oral transmission of knowledge and the necessity for each person to be in harmony with himself, his society and environment, as well as the spirit world. An individual is seen as inseparable from their milieu and the therapeutic approach is designed to address the body, mind, spirit, and emotions within the social and environmental context.

The milieu of a person includes the legends and myths of their culture.[1] These are significant because they tell of events that have become central to their sense of self and identity. It is while listening to such stories that a person can internalise and process the many messages they impart. The legends tell us of The Tuatha de Danann and their mythical god of healing called Déin Chécht, who had a son, Miach, and a daughter, Airmed, who were also healers. The legends tell us of the significance of psycho-somatic illness and the means used to address and cure it. Medicinal baths, cupping, surgery, as well as the use of sound give a glimpse of a therapeutic repertoire that was comprehensive and wide-ranging.

In Ireland, the coming of Christianity led to the indigenous belief system being syncretised with the new faith as well as a blossoming of literacy. The old gods dimmed and were replaced by Patrick and Colmcille, but the goddess Brigid remained and obtained her own feast day on February 1st. She was, and is, the guardian of the hearth of the home, whereas Mary, the mother of God, is relegated to the gables. The gables are external, but the hearth is where the fire of love, sustenance, and renewal resides. Brigid's association with fertility, as well as her role as the triune goddess of healing, poetry, and smithcraft, ensured her continued central presence in the daily lives of the people.

The healing modalities during these centuries centre on the miracles of the saints, the importance of relics and, as always in Ireland, pilgrim journeys to sacred spaces. The law tracts, *Bretha Crólige* and *Bretha Déin Chécht** dating from the eight century, tell us about the compensation due in the event of injury and the laws relating to the maintenance of a sick person, whereas *The Annals*† record the various plagues and pestilences that ravaged the country at various times. There is not much detail about therapeutics from this period, but the detail of terms given regarding a health issue, such as piles for example, is impressive and suggests careful observation of change and pattern in an illness.

Ireland has a treasure trove of medical manuscripts and the compilation and translation of these was undertaken in the medical schools, which were organised and regulated by the hereditary medical families. These manuscripts are, mainly, adaptations or translations into Irish, of European Latin treatises. One of these translations and compilations, *An Irish Materia Medica,* was completed by Tadgh Ó Cuinn in 1415 and serves as a useful base point to discuss the origin of herb use today. It is all too easy to forget that knowledge has no borders and the Irish hereditary medical families were part of a broader intellectual network of professionals[3] and students who travelled to Europe to keep up to date with contemporary medical knowledge.

Immigrants to Ireland from the 17th century had herbals in the English language available to them. Some these of these were Culpeper's written in London in 1653, Threkeld's written in Dublin in 1725, and that of K'Eogh in Cork in 1736. By comparing herbals written in the 20th century with these older books it is possible to establish, to some extent, where the information regarding the current use of a herb originates. Instances of such provenance are illustrated in Table 1 and Table 2.

Authors such as Lady Gregory and Wilde at the end of the 19th century and early 20th century give us an insight into the vernacular understanding of illness. We see, through their eyes, that illness could be caused by the "Sí," with the evil eye, the fairy dart and the changeling falling under this designation. The National Folklore Collections (NFC and NFCS) serve as a portal to the practice and opinion of Irish indigenous medicine in the 1930s. Again, the attributes of indigenous

---

*Also spelt as *Dianchecht.*
†The Annals of Ireland by the Four Masters, usually shortened to "The Annals."

medicine as it is understood in the global context are clearly evident in this magnificent collection.

Chapter 3 explores the possible causes of decline in the acceptance and practice of vernacular medicine. There were several factors in the 19th century that helped to erode a traditional way of life in many areas. One of these was the establishment of a national primary educational system where the medium of teaching was English. Further research will unravel the importance of "the grandmother factor" in this loss, and Gearóid Ó Tuathaigh has already highlighted this potential research area in relation to the loss of the Irish language and the inter-generational discord this must have engendered.[4] The potato famine of the 1840s, and the resulting increase in emigration, did nothing to lessen the destruction of the traditional way of life. Larkin[5] has also stressed the significance of the rising power of the Roman Catholic church for the widespread adoption of Victorian mores, as this suited the ambitions of the rising middle class in the country. More significantly is a point, the historian, Kwasi Konadu[6] makes about a colonised people, namely, that even on winning their independence they will only value what the coloniser valued, and associate anything demeaned or ignored by the coloniser as not worthy of development or preservation. Irish literature and music were valued, vernacular medicine was not.

Finally, in Chapter 4 I try to show how aspects of Irish indigenous medicine may be incorporated into a person's life today. By following the seasons of the year, we are able to connect with the Irish medical tradition and include it in daily life. This can be achieved through rituals, pilgrimage, and visits to sacred spaces, all of which helps us to realise that we are immersed in a sacred and therapeutic landscape, if we take the time to integrate it into our lives.

CHAPTER 1

What is medicine?

Our understanding of health and illness, as well as the means to maintain and treat it, is mediated by the culture in which we live and the ideas that inform that culture. The practical and functional choices people make about healthcare, and the practices they choose to use alongside conventional biomedicine, are formed from their own observations and "from the shared, often tacit, rules and values"* of their society.[7] How people see and understand things depends, not only on the worldview of the larger society in which we live, but also on any social grouping to which we belong within that society, be it a trade union, political party, religious affiliation, or sports club. These beliefs, and the concepts that inform them, form the basis of the knowledge and skills people need and use in daily life, including those used for the, "maintenance of health as well as the prevention, diagnosis, improvement or treatment of physical and mental illness."†[8]

---

*Bonnie Blair O'Connor, *Healing Traditions: Alternative Medicine and the Health Professions* (Philadelphia: University of Pennsylvania 1995), 7.
†WHO Traditional Medicine Strategy 2014-2023. World Health Organisation. Accessed 07/30/2021. https://www.who.int/publications/i/item/9789241506096;

The core elements of any medical system are diagnosis, prognosis, treatment, and prevention of ill health. These core elements do not change, but the medical systems which give them expression may evolve, mutate, and even die, because their fortunes are tied up with the changing cultural, technological, and economic paradigms of their societies. Biomedicine* is the main healing system in the western world and is becoming ever more reliant on technology and pharmaceutical expertise. Traditional Chinese medicine in Asia, Ayruveda in India, and Unani, and its variants, in the Arab world, South Africa, and India are other medical systems that have documented histories going back thousands of years with their knowledge being enlarged and refined over the centuries. As well as these great scribal traditions, there are the medical practices of indigenous people where the knowledge is passed on orally, by clearly defined teaching paths, to each succeeding generation. Generally, we examine other medical paradigms through the lens of scientific medicine and with the same conceptual tools,[9–11] but Alver and Selberg[9] suggest that examining indigenous medicine from the viewpoint of scientific medicine is inadequate and that it needs to be explored within the worldview of the culture that has generated it.

This book is about Irish indigenous medicine, and the worldview that informs this medical paradigm still permeates Irish culture forming the warp and weft of our daily living, even though we are, for the most part, unaware of its value and significance.

The Irish are not generally seen as an indigenous people similar to the Native Americans or Inuit of Canada, but have, like indigenous people elsewhere, suffered the effects of colonisation and land dispossession, as well as the historic injustices relating to their culture that stem from this.[12] Therefore, to understand the riches of the Irish indigenous medical tradition we need to explore how and why it differs from biomedicine and how, instead, it shares many characteristics and worldviews with traditional and indigenous medicine elsewhere. We have to try and understand why this intangible cultural heritage, this forgotten treasure trove of healing practices, that is to be found in the legends, *The Annals* medical manuscripts, and the National Folklore Collections,

---

*Modern western scientific medicine is called biomedicine because it explains health in terms of biology. It attaches importance to understanding the underlying physiology of the body. It uses diagnostic and laboratory-based testing to establish what is wrong and then repairs it. The biomedical model is the way healthcare is perceived in Western cultures.

is not lauded and feted throughout the land at this present time. At the core of my exploration, of Ireland's hidden medicine, is the premise that our understanding of health and illness, as well as the means to maintain and treat it, is mediated by the culture in which we live and the beliefs and opinions that inform that culture.

The choices people make about healthcare, and the practices they choose to use alongside conventional biomedicine, are constructed from their own observations and experience, as well as a shared understanding of the tacit rules and values within their society.[7] Acupuncture will not be a therapeutic choice for a person whose social circle has never heard of it, but it will be for a person whose social group includes it within their medical options as a valid therapeutic possibility.

People's health choices are, usually, pragmatic even though the cultural theories that inform a person's choice of treatment may not be understood. Acupuncture, for example, is based on the belief in Chinese medicine that there are energy channels throughout the body that can be activated to maintain health and heal illness. Western biomedicine does not believe in the existence of such channels, yet the use of acupuncture for the treatment of health issues has increased exponentially in the West. This increase would not have happened if people did not experience the positive effects of acupuncture in relieving health problems. This positive experience has allowed acupuncture to become one of the realistic and feasible choices people now make when they evaluate their healthcare options, even though the theories and belief system that inform this treatment modality lie very firmly in the worldview and philosophy of Chinese culture—a philosophy not necessarily understood by many patients receiving acupuncture. Different cultures, then, give rise to different perceptions of medicine and there are two main types in the world today: biomedicine and traditional medicine.

Biomedicine is a more accurate term to describe modern Western medicine, and the scientific basis that underpins biomedicine discounts the inherent complexity of the emotional/intellectual/physical/spiritual entity that is man. It puts enormous value on scientific methods of discovery and its treatment methodology is based on the body's biological systems. It has built its expertise, diagnostic methods, and therapeutics, on an understanding of the biology of man, and the effects that different factors, such as genetics, bacteria, and viruses, have on his biological makeup. In biomedicine, if the problem is affecting a particular biological system, such as pneumonia affecting the respiratory system, the problem can be identified, isolated, treated, and the person restored to health. The specific illness or organ is the problem and is perceived as a discrete entity to the person as a whole. This is at variance with other medical systems where allowance is made for the effect of personal, social, economic, and environmental factors in ill health, rather than concentrating solely on an isolated organ. This specialized approach of biomedicine contrasts with the constitutional method of diagnosis* present in Greek medicine, a method which prevailed in Europe up to the advent of modern scientific methods that occurred during the 18th century.

Traditional medicine includes medical traditions other than biomedicine and may be divided into two. The first branch includes the well-documented traditions of Chinese, Ayurvedic, and Greek/Unani medicine, and the second branch comprises the oral medical traditions of indigenous communities. Indigenous medicine is the term used to describe the range of healing methods used by any indigenous community, be they the Native Americans, African, South American, Australian, or Canadian indigenous peoples. These healing practices have developed empirically, are confined to a particular people, and are transmitted orally to each generation by a defined learning process. Even though there are common characteristics within the worldwide range of indigenous medicine, each community's medicine will be unique and will depend on local beliefs and environment.[13–15] The Inuit of Canada will not have expertise in healing snake bites nor the Navajo from Arizona in healing frostbite. Turning to Ireland, our indigenous medicine is often referred to as traditional or folk medicine but the most common description one hears from many people is, "he (or she) has a cure." These practitioners are, usually, not well known, have different therapeutic practices, operate on word-of-mouth recommendation, and are not governed by any specific legal statute or professional regulation. Biomedicine, on the other hand, is the system on which the Irish state's

---

*Hippocratic or Greek medicine attributes four elements to man, as making up the constitution of man. These are earth, air, fire, and water. Any combination of these determines a person's constitutional type and this has an influence on the illnesses he experiences. A person with too much water may be prone to respiratory illnesses and may also carry too much weight and be lazy. A person with too much fire may be of fiery nature and may be prone to skin or cardiovascular problems. If the different elements in a person are in balance, then the individual will be healthy, if not, he becomes ill. Diagnosis and treatment in this tradition is based on understanding this imbalance in the body and restoring it.

healthcare system is based, and it is governed by a comprehensive system of professional regulation and law.

What is the difference between these two systems of medicine, namely, the cures, charms, prayers, and rituals associated with the Irish healing tradition, and modern biomedicine with its vast array of technological expertise? The difference can be traced to the belief system embedded in each of these traditions, because these beliefs affect how illness is perceived, diagnosed, and treated. Both belief systems are present in Ireland. The belief system informing biomedicine originated in theories developed over four hundred years ago.

The biomedical model

Up to the late Middle Ages, people saw life holistically. Christianity permeated their worldview wherein the purpose of man's life was to achieve eternal life through good living. In the 14th century, Thomas Aquinas wedded Aristotelian thought with Christian theology, a union that provided a synthesis of reason and faith. Man is able to reason and because of this he can know and understand the world around him. However, the knowledge thus accrued is not innate but is gained through his senses. It is through his experience of the material world and reflection on his observations and experiences that man acquires knowledge and wisdom. Questions about God, ethics, social values, the human soul, and spirit are not only valid, but valued, as they lead to a greater understanding of man's place in the universe. Man and his relationship with the world around him is not only important, but central to his understanding of himself, nature, and society.

Aristotelian thought also influenced medicine with the Greek medical tradition being systematized by Hippocrates in the 4th century BC and developed further by Dioscorides (40–90 AD) and Galen (129-c200/c216 AD) in later centuries. Even though the Roman Empire fell to the onslaught of barbarian invasions, Greek medicine continued to be developed by, among others, Persian physicians such as Rhazes (854–925) and Avicenna (980–1037). It is now known as the Unani tradition and is still widely practised in Persia, Pakistan, India, South Africa, and (to a lesser extent) England.

When the medical community at Salerno, Montpelier, and Bologna first introduced Galenic medicine in the 11th and 12th centuries, it was a movement away from the more empirical approach being practised up to then. This change from the empirical to the theoretical was brought about by the presence of a strong medical community in Salerno from the 950s AD, as well as the importance of the Abbey of Montecassino near the city as a centre of translation. One of the monks at Montecassino, Constantine the African,* a translator *par excellence*, translated important Arabic and Greek texts into Latin. Even though these translations were undertaken in the latter half of the 11th century, research scientist Marco Valussi, in his insightful work on the European medieval medical system, maintains that their significance was not appreciated by the community of physicians in Salerno until the middle of the 12th century, over fifty years later.[16] The discovery of this corpus of knowledge had important consequences, as it fused the rational analysis of Aristotle with Galenic medicine and consequently transformed medicine. From this time on, medicine became more conceptualised, and the physician, through the humoral theory, was able to examine the relationship of man (microcosm) with the world around him (macrocosm). Among this body of learning was the *Al Qanun Fi Al-Tibb* (The Canon of Medicine) by the Persian physician Avicenna, and this became the standard medical text of European universities until the mid-17th century, as well as giving rise to the university-trained physician.

Also, in the sixteenth and seventeenth centuries people began to see the world, and their place in it, differently. This change in peoples' worldview was brought about by the ideas and theories proposed and promulgated during this era; ideas which gained considerable traction and acceptance over the following decades, as well as being developed, honed, and refined. These ideas form the basis of Western culture today, including its medicine.

The world-famous physicist Fritjof Capra sees this change from a holistic worldview to a mechanistic one, a change which also includes medicine, commencing with the heliocentric theory of Copernicus (1473–1543).[17] This theory made the sun, not the earth, the centre of the universe, a view totally opposed by the church of the time. Galileo (1564–1642) advocated this theory also and fell foul of the Church inquisition as a result. Isaac Newton (1642–1726), who was born the year Galileo died, copper fastened the heliocentric theory in 1687 and explained comprehensively why the planets moved around the sun and

---

*Died before 1098/1099.

how gravity was the force that kept them in check.* Earth was no longer the centre of the universe, but simply a small planet circling the sun.

However, Galileo is more famous because of his realisation that the laws of nature are, essentially, mathematical and can be solved through mathematical principles. In practice this meant that only the properties of objects that could be measured and quantified were worthy of study. Any subjective experience of an object, of its taste, smell, beauty, or aesthetic appreciation, did not count as they could not be measured mathematically. This view marked a significant step in the separation of science from religion and philosophy and reduced the status of the latter two.

While Galileo (1564–1642) was kicking up a storm in Italy advocating the role of mathematics in solving the mysteries of the universe, René Descartes (1596–1650) was doing the same in France, where he advocated the use of scepticism and reason in solving any problem. Like Galileo, Descartes posited that the language of nature was mathematics and that nothing can be proven to be true unless it can be described with the clarity of a mathematical demonstration. One's subjective experience was not important, not even relevant, because it could be inaccurate. This approach to knowledge blew the Aristotelian/Thomistic empirical approach to knowledge out the window, including the importance and centrality of man, a situation from which he has not yet recovered.

Descartes[18] was a formidable, if peripatetic, scholar and may justifiably be called the father of the scientific method. His greatest achievement was the development of analytical geometry,† and the concepts he developed are still indispensable in mathematics and other sciences. His influence is still felt in our lives because we still solve problems in the way he approached them. A problem should be divided and broken up into as many parts as possible and then arranged in a logical order. This logical arrangement is linear by default as one tests each thought and idea starting with the simplest, building and ascending

---

*The three laws of motion that Newton developed in his work laid the foundation for classical mechanics and contributed to many of the advances that occurred during the industrial revolution that followed a short time later.
†Descartes' analytical geometry was a tremendous conceptual breakthrough, linking the previously separate fields of geometry and algebra. Descartes showed that he could solve previously unsolvable problems in geometry by converting them into simpler problems in algebra. He represented the horizontal direction as x and the vertical direction as y. This concept is now indispensable in mathematics and other sciences.

little by little, and step by step, to more complex knowledge. Finally, the records kept of this process are so complete that nothing is omitted, and a complete understanding of the issue is acquired. An interesting, if not ironic, point about Descartes's scientific method, the cornerstone of which is mathematical certainty, is that these insights came to him in a series of dreams in November 1619. Being a devout Catholic, he attributed these dreams to a spirit sent from God to help him[18] (a fact that most certainly could not be assessed with mathematical certainty).

Descartes was methodical and analytical in his approach to a problem and considered that it was possible to discover the basic mechanical principles of natural phenomena and "thus render ourselves the lords and possessors of nature."[19] His philosophy introduced a separation of body and spirit, since anything to do with the spirit, including his dreams, cannot be analysed with mathematical certainty. Even if our body-machine is complex, it can ultimately be broken down into its component parts, which can then be examined to ascertain the truth. This division has led us to think of our minds as being "inside" our bodies and to viewing our bodies as something external to the "real" us, rather than viewing ourselves as an organic whole.

Like Descartes, Englishman Francis Bacon (1561–1626) was similarly critical of the scholastic tradition and believed that science was the key to technological progress. He also suggested that true objective knowledge could be built up through successive steps, where one starts with a lesser maxim and when that is proved correct one moves on to the next, and so on, until the last and most general knowledge is achieved. Each step of the way must be proven correct before the next stage is examined. The same inductive, progressive, and cumulative method is still used in science today, whereby a hypothesis is tested for its validity and each subsequent hypothesis is built on the previous one. We ignore questions that may side-track us in our step-by-step approach to our solution. The aim and work of science, for these scholars, was not integration with the world but domination of it. Earth was no longer a living organism but a machine that could be used according to man's will.

The two hundred years from Copernicus to Newton was a period of incredible change, a period where the old theories, such as those of Ptolemy in Geography, Aristotle in Physics, and Galen in medicine, were superseded. New concepts formed the foundation for the scientific achievements that were to follow, and have followed, to the present day. Descartes and Bacon considered scepticism and doubt to be essential to the scientific endeavour. They believed that the person searching after truth must always remember that man's observation may be illusory. Good examples of which would be the common belief that the sun rotates around the earth, or that the earth was flat. This contrasted with the old Aristotelean premise that our perception and cognitive faculties are reliable. It follows, from this distrust of man's own observations, that anything that cannot be measured mathematically was of no interest to science as it was not verifiable. This ruled out a person's emotional and spiritual knowledge as having any scientific value as these are largely subjective.

The consequent influence of this way of thinking on medicine was remarkable as, coupled with advances in technology, it allowed a person's body to be objectified, examined, and treated independently of his or her environment. To science, a kidney is a kidney no matter where the person lives. Man's circulatory system is the same the world over, as is his liver. Each organ and biological system can be treated without reference to a person's individual circumstances, his environment, his socio-economic status, or his culture. Western medicine sees illness as a biological* or pathological phenomenon, including psychiatric illness,[20] and if no physiological or biochemical abnormality can be identified in the organ affected, the possibility of a psychosomatic disorder is considered. This is a psychological condition that manifests as physical symptoms that lack a direct pathological or biological cause. Functional somatic syndromes (FSS), are often a result of psychosomatic disorders and they present with a variety of different signs and symptoms.[21] If a patient is diagnosed with functional somatic syndrome, there will often be a history of physical complaints, an impairment of functioning, medical interventions, but ultimately there is a lack of explanation, on any obvious organic level, for the reported symptoms or their severity. As FSSs can manifest in various areas of the body,† a different specialist will be consulted depending on the most prominent symptom. If fibromyalgia is present, the rheumatologist is the consultant of choice; the gastroenterologist if abdominal pain with altered bowel habits is present,

---

*The biomedical model refers to the dominant medical system in the industrial world, which is based on biological investigations of disease at the molecular level.

†The term "functional somatic syndrome" describes a combination of symptoms that cannot be fully explained by pathological conditions or diseases. However, they cause disruption of everyday activities and may lead to an endless round of medical investigations with no conclusive result.

and chronic fatigue and myalgia becomes a post-viral or chronic fatigue syndrome for the infectious-diseases specialist.[21] Even though FSS may have emotional, spiritual, and other non-verifiable causes, biomedicine does not currently have the tools to address them.

There is one other important concept that Europeans have inherited from Aristotle, and that is the concept of the uncaused cause or the Prime mover. In simple terms, Aristotle accepted that everything in the world is constantly changing, be it the movement of the planet or steam turning to water. He argued that this constant movement could not have come about by itself but must have been brought about by something that is itself unmoved, that is not caused by any prior action. He called this the Prime Mover, Thomas Aquinas called it God and for Lao Tzu, the great Chinese philosopher, it was Tao.[22] Even though Aristotelian and Christian thought accepts that the Prime Mover may be recognized as imminent within, and manifest in creation, it is commonly perceived as being transcendent, above and beyond the universe, like a clockmaker winding up a clock. Similarly, in Chinese thought, Tao is the source of all existence, the root of all things, but the way to understand the Tao is to observe the patterns within the universe and follow nature's direction. It is by doing this that all creatures will prosper. So, though at first sight Aristotle's idea of a Prime Mover may seem irrelevant to us, this is not so, as it creates a linear pattern with God at the apex and mud at the bottom. This Great Chain of Being ranks all beings in an ascending order from the inanimate world to other animals and then to humans. Above man are angels and finally, God, the unmoved Mover. This divinely ordained chain of being was very useful politically as it validated the feudal system with the king at the top and the serf at the bottom, but this linear chain also encouraged man to see himself as a conqueror of nature, apart and separate from it.

This concept of a Prime Mover also means that Europeans, generally look for the cause when something happens, rather than the form or pattern within what is happening. A simple example of a river in flood will illustrate how this concept may not work in everyday life. If a river is overflowing, the pattern or attributes of the river will be more important than the cause. A flood that is strong rapid and turbulent will necessitate a different response to a slow-moving body of water with no great force other than volume. The cause of the flood may be a burst dam or torrential rain, but this cause cannot be separated from the pattern or form of the flood and how this needs to be addressed. The work of Descartes, Galileo, and Bacon all stemmed from the need to know the cause, and this has continued to the present day. In terms of illness, it means we concentrate on the cause of the illness rather than the movement or pattern of the illness itself. By looking for a cause for illness external to the individual we are again able to divorce the illness from the person. This way of thinking has removed the social and environmental aspects of healing as well as a therapeutic approach based on the pattern of the illness. The Cartesian belief that man can become masters of nature has also been fed by this linear way of thinking, and technology has added fuel to this particular fire by enabling science to learn more and more about the mechanics of objects, be it the kidney, the blood, the grass, or the soil. This way of thinking is in direct contrast with the indigenous worldview.

The indigenous model

There is the mistaken assumption that before the re-introduction of Hippocratic and Galenic medicine into Europe there was no medicine or medical facilities.[23] This is an erroneous assumption, as man has always sought to heal and has developed many ways to do that depending on his environment. Within Europe there has always been a folk medicine, even though it was generally seen as representing a "little culture" vis a vis the "larger culture" of formal systems of medical education.[24] Many of the medicines that are basic to biomedicine, such as metformin derived from Galega officinalis, and digoxin from Digitalis lanata, originated in folk medicine. It is also incorrect to assume that there was a great gap between the university-trained physician and the many other types of healers who practised before the advent of the formal academic training to qualify as a doctor. It was the latter that led, in the 12th–13th centuries, to the stratification of medical practitioners with the university graduate physician occupying the topmost point in the hierarchy.[16] Up to this, civil authorities licensed doctors to practise medicine without a university degree and definitions of what a doctor was were very fluid. All practitioners worked in an overlapping market and belonged to a continuum of care ranging from domestic medicine for chronic conditions to professional medicine for acute situations.[25]

Within indigenous communities knowledge, generally, can be grouped into four broad areas: oral tradition, a quotidian awareness of the spirit world, a close connection with nature, and a living repository of stories that create a sense of identity and meaning.[26] These four characteristics are also present in Ireland;

The oral tradition in Ireland is evident in the way knowledge was transmitted to the next generation and included the practical skills of everyday living, as well as the knowledge and skills associated with specific occupations, such as currach making, iron work, and textile production. People living in an indigenous agricultural society will view the world differently to someone living in an urban environment, not least in their sense of time. When life revolves around the growing and harvesting of food, time will be perceived as unfolding in a cyclical manner rather than linear. The waxing and waning of the moon, the lengthening and shortening of the day is what will govern daily life. The unfolding year, as well as nature both in its benign and harsh aspects, assumes importance, with different signs in nature being observed to see if they are for good or ill. Life rotates around what is observed, and experienced, and daily life is part of the endless cycle of birth, growth, and decay. There is a familiarity with the energy of the earth, that gives life to all creatures including man. The rush of energy in the spring suffusing the entire landscape and the quietude of the winter when no growth can be seen tell that the earth is a living being with its own rhythm and cyclical activity. It is no wonder then that when the chieftain was elected by the *deirfinn*, his enthronement ceremony included a mystical marriage to the earth, for whom he was, as chieftain, to care. If the fertility of the earth declined or plague ravaged the kingdom, he could be executed for not fulfilling this duty.

Farming teaches through experience. Each year brings new knowledge, and this heritage is transmitted orally to the next generation. This transmission is not erratic or sporadic but is, instead, carefully structured according to gender, capability, and age.[27] A child of three will not be taught how to plough a field, but he will be shown the plough and tackle. He will see his father tackle the horse, his relationship with the animal, his care, or his cruelty. All this he will learn, and, unlike book knowledge, he will interiorise it. Book knowledge would separate him from the lived experience. No diagram in a book could capture the work worn hands of his father caressing the harness as he slips it over the back and head of the horse. No written instruction could capture the time taken in the waxing and oiling of the harness to ensure no chafing for the animal and to ensure longevity for the tackle.

Spirituality, and acknowledgement of nature as gift, is intrinsic to the beliefs of indigenous communities.[24] spirituality, in this sense, is not only the subjective experience of a sacred dimension, but is also inclusive of a spirit world, an otherworld.[28] In the late 19th and early 20th century, accounts by Wilde,[29] Gregory[30] and Wood Martin[31] attest to a strong belief in the existence of the otherworld in contemporary Ireland, "a domain relating to the preternatural, an alternative realm parallel to or sometimes beyond human earthly existence,"[32] a belief that was commonplace in all parts of the country and in all levels of society. These spirits may or may not impinge upon the human world. Evidence of the awareness of this spirit world in everyday life is to be found in the many rituals and stories associated with the "good people", who co-existed alongside the world of mortals[32] and who were "everywhere around us" with "the power to go in every place."[33]

The otherworld may be observed in expressions of popular belief and practice, such as the importance of luck, time and space, as well as acceptance of individuals with extraordinary powers. It is also seen in the tolerant, and open-minded attitude towards charms, divination, the fairies, emblems, numbers and colours, and much more.[34] Spirituality can also be inferred from the mythological tradition, where belief in the devil, supernatural beings, and demons is evident. The importance of the world of the spirit, and the importance of keeping balance between the worlds, may also be seen in the traditions associated with nature, such as the religious traditions and festivals, as well as the four-fold division of the Irish calendar year—*Samhain, Imbolc, Bealtaine* and *Lughnasa*.

The close connection with nature is evidenced by the annual cycle of rituals associated with the seasons and the cycle of food production. The expression of community skill in music, dance, and oral literature also added meaning to the unfolding year, and affirmed the cyclical nature of the seasons and close community ties.[35]

The *Leabhar Gabhála Érenn*/The Book of Invasions supplies the "origin story" for the people of the island; medieval scholars regarded this story as a standard part of Irish history and recorded it as such. Legends recounted in Ireland tell of kings, wars, and heroes, but may also include tales of buried treasure, ghosts, fairies, and saints.[36] In an indigenous society, knowledge is accrued through observation, experience, and utility and is stored in people's memories and activities, including a community's stories, songs, folklore, proverbs, dance, myth, cultural values, beliefs, and rituals.[10, 37, 38] As life is governed by daylight, the long winter evening are times to set apart to tell and hear the stories of their race. How they came to this island, and how their forebears were responsible for wondrous deeds. The child thus learns that he belongs to a great race of gods and fighting men. He learns of Brigit of the Gael to whom the heart of the house belongs. Mary, the mother of God, keeps the gables safe but the heart of the home belongs to Brigit. She is the triune goddess of poetry, healing, and metal work; so great a goddess that Christianity acknowledged her as a saint, giving her *Imbolc*, February 1st, as her saints day. Brigid is the protector of the hearth, that primeval flame that gives warmth to man and separates him from the beast in the field who seeks shelter among the trees and hedgerows.

Indigenous medicine has been viewed as a historic phenomenon, and studies pertaining to it have used the framework and concepts of scientific biomedicine to examine its effectiveness.[9] However, this framework and these concepts are inadequate for any examination of vernacular healing practices, including those evident in Irish vernacular medicine.[6, 13, 20, 39] An indigenous medicine is born from the worldview of the community and has certain characteristics. In illustrating some of these I will refer mainly to Ireland, where it is still practised, even though we have inherited both an oral and Galenic tradition. The indigenous oral Irish medical tradition, until the fall of the Gaelic order, was in the hands of hereditary medical families with the physician being under the patronage of the chief of the locality. Their only duty was to maintain the health of the people and they were given land, the rent of which allowed them to concentrate on their medical practice. Laws relating to the oral tradition may be found in the *Bretha Crólige*, and the *Bretha Déin Chécht*, which date from the 8th century.[40, 41] According to the *Bretha Déin Chécht*, there are three errors in the care of a patient, namely, lack of nursing and medical care, lack of a suitable diet, and the failure to provide an income for the dependents of the sick patient.[42] Moreover, physicians from this tradition went abroad to Montpellier and Salerno to learn about the new Galenic tradition being taught there and introduced this knowledge to Irish medical schools between 1400 and 1700. These European sojourns resulted in a large corpus of medical writing, in Irish, giving an account of Galenic medicine in Ireland in late medieval and early modern Ireland.[43] This hereditary medical system disappeared with the passing of the old Gaelic order* in the early 17th century.

Medicine within indigenous cultures displays many of the same characteristics as biomedicine today, even if at first glance this does not appear to be so. Firstly, there is the diviner who may be seen as parallel to the general practitioner (GP) in that he divines/diagnoses what the problem is. Where the GP uses instruments, such as stethoscope, ophthalmoscope, and otoscope, the diviner may use twigs off a tree, the pattern of stones, or dream interpretation to identify the cause of the malaise. If the diviner considers he has the competence and skills to treat you, just like a GP, he will do so. If not, he will refer you to the most appropriate healer among the indigenous health care professionals. In Ireland, these are the *bean ghlúine*, the *bean* or *fear feasa/leighis* and the physical therapist.

The midwife was known as the *bean ghlúine*, and the diviner, spiritualist, and plant medicine man were often seen in the one person, known as the *bean feasa/leighis* meaning wise/healer. Ó Crualaoich maintains, "that the power of these women to diagnose and minister ... was held to derive from their close association with the native otherworld and the knowledge and skill which that association conferred.†[44] There is one other person in the Irish medical panel, leaving aside the bonesetter, and that is the *bean caointe*. Her job was to *caoin*‡ at the wake and funeral, but one may say she is now replaced by the eulogy.

Where belief in the preternatural is an integral part of a people's worldview, this will also permeate any understanding of medicine. In an international context, different scholars,[13][45–51] have identified illnesses believed to be of preternatural origin as an integral component

---

*The Gaelic political and social order, and its associated culture, that existed in Ireland from the prehistoric era until the early 17th century. Before the Norman invasion of 1169, Gaelic Ireland comprised the whole island. Thereafter, it comprised that part of the country not under foreign dominion at a given time.

† Gearóid Ó Crualaoich, *The Book of the Cailleach* (Cork: Cork University Press), 72.

‡ The following is a description of the "Caoining" ... The four "Caoiners" took up their positions, two on each side of the corpse, the second day of the wake. They then started relating the dead person's good qualities, all the time crying and clapping their hands. Sometimes their voices were hushed to a whisper often raised to a shriek. This continued for a considerable time. Then one of them started a chant in a weird voice, the others at this time remaining silent. This chant was in some sort of rhyme and always was the subject of the dead person's ancestors, their great deeds either in battle, or their fame in hurling or other games. At intervals this chant ended in crying in which all four took part. NFCS 0382:075.

of indigenous medicine. Of these, Professor Ikechi Mgbeoji[13] cogently and clearly describes the importance of not separating the emotional and the spiritual from the physical in any healing modality: "As practitioners of a recognizable regime of healthcare, traditional healers operate from a worldview that construes ailment and disease as a psychosomatic phenomenon, rather than a biological or pathogenic phenomenon."[13] Even though his discussion pertains to the Ngwa people of south eastern Nigeria only, his observations could, with geographical and cultural variations, be made relevant to indigenous medicine anywhere. This view is supported by other scholars, who all stress that illness may have a spiritual and emotional origin just as much as a physical one. Within Ireland, illnesses that were attributed to the sí are the evil eye, the fairy blast, the changeling, and "being taken by the fairies."

Today in Ireland, a practitioner of indigenous medicine is known as a "person with a cure." He or she may have a cure for eczema, TB, skin cancer, or haemorrhage. They come from all walks of life, and they have received their gifts by different means. There are various ways in which a person can receive the authority to heal, but the most common is that of lineage. Many healers of indigenous medicine can trace their lineage back nine or ten generations. The Lanes, the bonesetters currently practising in north Cork, are probably descended from the hereditary medical family called the Ó Leighins who practised in much the same area, before the fall of the Gaelic order, in the early part of the 17th century. In the Elizabethan fiants* of 1640, there are sixteen people mentioned with the name Ó Leighin and the occupation of fifteen of these is entered as chirosurgeon. The occupation of the sixteenth is that of "seargeant," which may well be a misrepresentation of the word surgeon.

There are other ways also to receive the authority to practise as a healer. One may be given a cure by somebody who already has it, but the stress here is on, "given the cure." You cannot ask for it, and I am familiar with the anguish of sons and daughters who have seen the family cure being given to someone outside the family, who did not value it, and subsequently never practised it. Usually, the healer will think long and carefully before they pass on a cure, as the person receiving it must

---

*A fiant was a writ issued to the Irish Chancery mandating the issue of letters patent. These published written orders were issued under the Great Seal of Ireland, and they covered areas such as appointments, government activities, and grants of pardon to the Irish.

understand that it is a gift and not charge for its use. To accept a cure is to accept responsibility. A cure may also be obtained by esoteric means, such as licking a lizard as a small child and subsequently having the ability to heal burns—if you lick the burn.[52] Being the seventh son of a seventh son and being a member of certain families, such as Cahills or Keoghs, also entitles you to practise as a healer for specific conditions. Having the same name as your partner on marriage is another way of acquiring a cure but in Co. Meath this is further constrained by the necessity to share the same Christian initial as well as surname.

It is only by acquiring the cure in a clearly defined way that one is qualified to practise. How the cure is transmitted or taught to the designee varies. Generally, those who use plant medicine have been taught from a young age, usually three to five.

Sean Boylan from Co. Meath is a traditional healer of vernacular medicine and was helping his father weeding herbs at four years of age. Another healer in the south of Ireland was observing his uncle treating cancer lesions from a similar age. A well-known bonesetter was foraging for plants for poultices as a young child, and also remembers the plants being processed in a "bothy out the back." As these healers got older, the level of knowledge that they received increased, until gradually they were allowed practice on their own.

There are different types of cures in the Irish corpus, and they can be broadly divided into three: plant medicine, physical manipulation, and charms prayer and rituals.

Plant medicine

Many healers consider secrecy to be a condition of their receiving the cure, which means the formula goes to the grave with their owner if it is not passed on and accepted by the designee.[53] The owner of a plant cure will consider the character of their son or daughter before they transmit knowledge of the cure. If the son is too wild or looks as if he will not use the cure responsibly, they will defer telling him essential elements of the cure, such as the plants used, where to find them, or how to prepare them, so they become effective. This delay may well have fatal consequences, as it often takes the demise of the father before the son settles down. By then it is too late. This brings to mind another important aspect in the efficacy of plant medicine, which the person steeped in Western biomedicine does not understand. This factor is captured in the frequent question, "what herb is good for?," as if there is a magic bullet, a single herb that will solve a particular ailment. This question fails to recognise the enormous expertise of the indigenous healer. The healer must first and foremost know what plants to pick. It is rare that a healer will only use one plant, as this level of knowledge would be well-known within the community generally. Also, such knowledge is generally incorporated into the diet, such as the antimicrobial properties of thyme being used in stuffing, sauces etc. or eating nettle in the month of May, a time when the leaves are young, tender, palatable, and easily digestible. The dock leaf is the antidote to the nettle sting, and this is knowledge known to the vast majority of people in the community. The healer, therefore, has much greater knowledge than that of simples. His/her expertise lies, firstly, in knowing what plant to pick, the best place to pick it and when to pick it. He/she needs to know what part of the plant to use and how to prepare this part of the plant. Finally, he/she need to know how to process the formula, so it becomes an efficacious product. The indigenous healer is, in modern terms, a botanist, horticulturist, pharmacist, and doctor all rolled into one. The final aspect of the healer's training involves the administration of the formula, when, in the case of a cream or poultice, it is to be applied, or taken, if the cure is a "bottle."

The word "bottle" is often used by people seeking a cure. They are going to see the healer, who has a "bottle" and this, generally, may be seen as synonymous with the word "cure." There is, however, another type of bottle and this bottle is not a one based on plants but is of a more esoteric nature. The healer, who has such a bottle, may well have a line of cars on the road leading to the house on Sunday afternoon seeking their life-giving treasure. There will be strict instructions on how to take the liquid in the bottle after which the contents must be discarded in a place where no man walks.

Physical manipulation

The second division of cures in the Irish healing tradition is that of physical manipulation. This is generally perceived as bonesetting, but there is also a manipulative technique known as "raising the breastbone." Bonesetting is generally considered, even by its practitioners, to be the realigning of dislocated bones. No bonesetter today will realign a fracture due to better facilities and pain control for such a procedure in a hospital. Though this development is understandable, it means there is a loss of knowledge due to non-practice and the rich knowledge of the indigenous healer in relation to fractures will be lost. One bone-setter told me that the splint used in a fracture had to be ash and the branch picked for use as splint had to be approximately four inches in diameter. The inside was hollowed out after being sliced in two, so that the sapwood of the branch lay against the fractured bone. One imagines a branch wrapped around a fractured bone to be terribly painful, but care was taken to bevel back the ends of the splint so that they did not chafe against the skin. Other important knowledge regarding fractures is that bones take longer to heal in winter than in summer, so the splint was left on for ten weeks in winter and only six in summer. This practice concurs with the knowledge that vitamin D is needed to set bones and there is a dearth of that during the long dark winter in Ireland. Another interesting piece of information is that a woman who is menstruating will not heal as quickly as a woman whose fracture occurs at another time.

Raising the breast-bone is a procedure that involves three successive visits of approximately one hour, possibly longer in some cases. Even though this is a well-documented tradition in the National Folklore Collections, and was well known up to the 1950s, there are very few practitioners today. This technique, and even the concept, of "raising the breast-bone" has no parallel in biomedicine. It may be seen as a form of cupping but is actually quite different.

Charms, prayers, and rituals

The third area of therapeutics is that of charms, prayers, and rituals. By and large, these are deemed *piseogs* or superstitions. Yet, despite being viewed in such a disparaging way they survive and are sought after. Their efficacy to the 20th century rational mind lies in the placebo effect, but 21st century research would place them in the developing area of psychoneuroendocrinology, where the nervous, endocrine, and immune systems relate and interact with each other.

Charms are known all over Europe and may be divided into different classes, such as those for pains, good luck, protection from burning etc. Most charms are now Christianised even though Hull[54] traces the use of Irish charms back to the Irish legendry god of medicine, Déin Chécht, where in an Irish manuscript at St. Gall monastery, Switzerland a charm against various ailments is recorded; "May that be made whole whereon the salve of Déin Chécht goes. I put my trust in the salve which Déin Chécht left with his people."[54]

One of the most popular charms known throughout Europe is the one for stopping bleeding. Before the age of clocks and watches, this charm may have been a means of measuring how long pressure is needed to be kept on a bleeding wound for it to clot. But this is not the whole answer. One healer, who has a charm for stopping bleeding, has told me that he receives over 5000 telephone calls annually requesting him to say the charm. He will answer his phone 24/7 and he receives calls from as far away as the United States and India. What causes a person living in the USA to seek such help when reason tells us that it is hocus pocus? I know professional healthcare workers, as well as others, who will swear that this charm worked for them or their loved ones.

This brings me to another aspect of the healer's cure and that is luck. Most healers do not charge for their cure, but some may accept a donation. This could be a five euro note or a pot of jam. Either is acceptable. Others are adamant they will accept nothing. If a donation is insisted on by the patient, it is, generally, put aside and donated to a charity at Christmas or at some other significant time during the year. This insistence of the person receiving the cure to give a donation, where none is requested, hinges upon the idea of luck and the following accounts explain this.

A certain healer lived in West Cork in the early part of the 20th century. He gave his cures freely and refused to accept payment. However, his own financial circumstances suffered, a calf would die, a crop would be poor, a sale not so profitable. He spoke of his dilemma to the local parish priest who suggested that he continue giving his cure but to charge a shilling. He did so, and his luck changed for the better. Another healer told me he has no such experience, no negative consequences to his giving of the cure, but that he knows of a healer who, having said a charm for someone, becomes bereft of energy. This weakness and lethargy are so severe he has to stay in bed for a few days until his vigour returns.

This idea of luck also hinges on the reciprocal nature of gift so comprehensively discussed by the sociologist and anthropologist, Marcel Mauss.[55] He argues that a gift carries something of the giver, an unseen attribute. To give a gift in return, no matter how small, is to return that attribute to the giver. This argument of Mauss appears to be the basis of the parish priest's advice, to the healer in West Cork, to charge a shilling. A grandchild of that West Cork healer sought to follow in his grandfather's footsteps (who had died some years previously) and asked his aunt for the formulae for the cures. She refused saying, "No, there's no luck following it."

Other cures may involve a ritual, and this may include the requirement to return on a set number of days, or a prohibition on eating or drinking for a period of time. In the case of the cure for "heart-fever," the prescribed ritual is continued over three days and recipients of this cure have told me that the ritual gives a sense of calm and serenity as well as the ability to face the word again. The very name of this cure, "heart-fever," gives an indication of the problem. In today's language it would be called burn out, emotionally overwhelmed. It is the situation where an individual feels unable to cope with the demands of home and business. The "heart fever" ritual allows one to take time out. It is an acknowledgement to oneself and the healer that life has become just too much. Conversation is forbidden during the ritual, and this in itself is healing. A ritual, by its very nature, is a time apart. It has a beginning and an end and involves prescribed actions by the healer and the patron. It is timeless in that it takes you out of ordinary time and links you not only to your community, but to your forebears who passed on the cure. It places you at the centre of a ritual that heals and consoles in the present but whose origin is in the distant past. It may be described as a crossroads where different roles converge, and balance and equilibrium are to be found. It is shaped by preceding life events and informs subsequent actions.[56]

Rituals associated with water are even more obvious in their association with ancient belief systems, and pattern days are days dedicated to pilgrimages to holy wells.[53] Within their environs, the landscape, the prayers, and the sun-wise direction, all contribute to identity, be it of self, family, or community. To walk other than a *deiseal* (clockwise) is unlucky and may bring about bad luck. While, doing these rounds in a sunwise direction, people pray, after which a person may drink from the well and then fill a bottle with its water. This is brought home to be used for blessing crops, animals and humans when deemed to be needed, and on certain festivals of the calendar year. As well as visiting wells on specific days, people also visit wells if there is a need. These springs are reputed to have healing properties and are often known by the relevant part of the anatomy, such as *tobair na suil* for the well water that cures afflictions affecting the eye. It is not unusual to see a hawthorn tree next to the well and this will be festooned with pieces of material, rosary beads, beads, and other forms of amulets. Known as rag trees, these trees and wells offer an oasis of peace to people in need of healing. They are scattered throughout the country and the freshness of some of the material hanging on the branches attest to their continued use.

The combination of a hawthorn tree and a well is a potent manifestation of the indigenous worldview. A lone hawthorn tree is associated with the fairy/spirit world, and no one will cut one down in fear of the consequences. Modern roads have been rerouted so as to not disturb such trees. Wells have always been associated with life giving properties, a manifestation of the earth's energy and sustenance as well as places of pilgrimage for healing.[57]

Other rituals involve smoke, such as in a cure for ringworm. This involves the healer burning three pieces of wood until they smoulder. Holding the sticks in his hand (each one is about the size of a cigar), he moves them in an east west circular movement over the ringworm patches. While doing this, the healer prays his prayer/mantra, *sotte voce*. The affected person has to return on three consecutive days, but one woman told me that the ringworm is usually gone in two. Probably the most difficult type of ritual to understand is the cure for a sprain, where the healer prays quietly to him/herself while holding the affected ankle, after which the swelling disappears and the ankle can take full weight within an hour, if not less. Another difficult cure to believe is the cure for shingles. The ritual involves the healer pricking his finger and placing the blood drawn on the shingle lesion, while saying the prescribed prayers. Again, the patient returns three times, but not necessarily on consecutive days.

It can be seen that the concept of a person having a healing gift, even though they are not medically qualified in the usual sense of the term, is an accepted part of Irish society. As recently as February 27th, 2020, a newspaper published an article about a priest, Fr. Conlon. This priest has been in the healing ministry for twenty-five years and it was his uncle who told him he had the gift of healing and gave him the cures:

> His uncle Joe was the one who told him, he could heal, who himself was known for healing, mostly animals, but people too. He gave

me certain prayers and told me I had all the cures. He had a special cure for psoriasis, or eczema. Children would come to him and it would heal up.[58]

There is then, a rich array of healing modalities in Irish indigenous medicine and it is now opportune to explore the history of medicine in Ireland to enquire into their possible source.

CHAPTER 2

History of irish indigenous medicine

Legend and myth

The story of a society's indigenous medicine starts with its legends and myths as these give insights into some of the medical practices followed in apocryphal times. In Ireland, the *Lebor Gabála Érenn* (LGE) is the origin story of the Irish people and its development draws from different sources and traditions. These sources may be traced to the 7th century, and as well as recording the deeds and genealogies of its rulers and heroes, it also purports to trace the lineage of the Gaels from Egypt to Scythia to Spain* and finally to Ireland.[59] Ó Corráin[60] tells us that a great deal of the material in these genealogies and historical narratives, "is independently verifiable and, given the difficulties of transmission, extremely accurate."†

---

*For further detailed discussion of the *Lebor Gabála Érenn* see, John Carey (Ed) *Lebor Gabála Érenn: Textual History and Pseudohistory* (Dublin: Irish Texts Society, 2009).
†Ó Corráin, Donncadh. Creating the Past: The Early Irish Genealogical Tradition. (Belgium: *Peritia* (12), 1998), 207.

Hospitals and physicians

In the LGE, one place of significance mentioned is Eamhain Macha,* the capital of the ancient kings of Ulster, situated on the western side of the current city of Armagh. The history of Eamhain Macha spans over 4000 years, its most important period being the late Bronze/early Iron age. Queen Macha Mong Ruadh, the daughter of Aed Ruadh, established the first hospital in Ulster there and it was called *Broin Bhearg*.[61]

> There were indeed three houses in Evan in the time of Conor, namely the Soldier's Sorrow, the Crimson Branch, and the Red Branch. In the first of these were the sick, and thus it was called the house of the Soldier's Sorrow, from the sorrow and affliction caused by the anguish of their wounds and diseases.[62]

Although the legends and myths of the history of Ireland have no verifiable foundation, there are some interesting references to how people were administered (herbal) medicines that are likely to have been very real. One of the legendry peoples of Ireland were the Tuatha De Dannan, and their God of health was a physician called Déin Chécht.[63] Miach and Airmed were two of his seven children and were herbal physicians and surgeons also. Lugh†was a grandson of Déin Chécht and one example of the use of herbs is a story about his magic spear. This weapon thirsted for blood, and because of this insatiable blood lust, it was kept at rest, outside of battle, by steeping its head in a sleeping draught of pounded poppy leaves. The ability of the herb *Papaver somniferum* to induce rest and sleep is also captured in its Irish name, *codalian*, from *codal* or *cada* meaning sleep.[64]

Medicinal baths

The use of incantation and medicinal herbal baths is widespread across the world and there are examples of same in the Anglo-Saxon

---

*The Four Masters record the foundation of the Ulster capital as follows:
The Age of the World 4540 (660 B.C.). The first year of Macha in the sovereignty of Ireland after the death of Cimbaoth, son of Fintan. The Age of the World 4546. Macha Mongruadh.was slain by Reachtaidh Righdhearg. It was Macha that commanded the sons of Diothorba to erect the fort of Eamhain, that it might be the city of Ulster forever.
†After whom the month of August is named in Irish: *Lughnasa*.

Leech books. This form of treatment was used in Ireland at the first and second battles of Moytura over three thousand years ago. Déin Chécht, his two sons and his daughter, chanted incantations over a well named Sláine.* The mortally wounded soldiers were placed in the well and through the power of incantation uttered by the four physicians around the well they emerged fully healed and ready for battle the next day. The well became known as Loch Luibe† because Déin Chécht put every herb that grew in Ireland into it.[2]

Herbal baths are also mentioned on the occasion of the army of the king of Leinster being attacked by enemies with poisoned weapons. This poison resulted in certain death from the slightest wound. Before the next battle, the milk of one hundred and fifty white, hornless cows was poured into a bath. Once they received a wound during the battle, the soldiers were plunged into the bath and the poison was neutralised in this manner.[61]

In the tales of the Red Branch Knights, the physicians/*liaig* [leea] were under the direction of Fingin Faithliaig, King Concobar's physician, during times of battle. Fingin also used baths to heal the wounded, and these baths not only contained medicinal herbs but also the marrow of a great number of cows. Each physician carried a bag of medicaments slung from his waist and at the end of each day's battle they ministered to the wounded. This bag of medicaments was known as a *lés* and Joyce, in *A Smaller Social History of Ireland*, remarks that a *liaig* attempting to cure without his *lés* was like the companions of St Columba after his death … helpless.[63]

Humour and expertise

The legends tell us of great skill but also reveal a sense of humour. The following is one such amusing tale.

At the end of the battle of Moytura, the King, Nuada, lost his arm and with such a blemish he could not retain the office of King. Déin Chécht, with the help of Credne the brazier, had a prosthesis of silver made to replace Nuada's hand and this was made so skilfully that all the joints moved, and it was as supple as a real hand. However, it was not enough to maintain the kingship and a new king was

* *Sláine* is the Irish for health.
† *Luibh* is the Irish for herb.

invited to rule over them. The new king became a dictator and all the subjects suffered. At this point in the saga, Déin Chécht's son, Miach, and his daughter, Airmid, came to visit the deposed king, Nuada. There was a porter at the entrance who had only one eye. He asked the visitors who they were, and they replied, "*We are good doctors.*" He immediately challenged their skill by suggesting they give him a new eye. They proposed removing one of the eyes of his cat, who was sitting nearby, and giving it to him instead. He was delighted with this offer, and they duly did what they had promised. Unfortunately for the porter, the eye retained its cat like nature, and he subsequently tended to stay awake at night and sleep during the day.

The porter reported this medical success to Nuada, who commanded that they be brought to him. On entering, Miach and Airmid heard the king groaning and noticed that the wrist had festered where the silver prosthesis joined the arm. Miach asked, where was the amputated hand? He was told it had been buried a long time ago. Nevertheless, he dug it up, placed it to Nuada's stump and uttered an incantation over it, saying: "Sinew to sinew, and nerve to nerve be joined!" and he healed it in nine days and nights. The first three days he carried it against his side, and it became covered with skin. The second three days he carried it against his chest. The third three days he cast white wisps of black bulrushes after they had been blackened in a fire.[2]

The mention of nine and three days are important in myth, with the number nine being associated with knowledge and the number three with the triple spiral motif so prevalent in Celtic stone art. The different stages in the progression of the grafting process also appears to show an understanding of grafting, as the incantation moves from muscular regeneration to nerve regeneration and the skin being used is from the thigh (carrying it against his side), which is a usual place for harvesting partial thickness skin grafts.

Déin Chécht's jealousy

Déin Chécht was jealous of Miach's superior surgery and struck his son's head with a sword. The blow was superficial and only cut the flesh. Miach healed it easily. Déin Chécht struck again, and this time cut through to the bone. Again, his son healed it, and this so enraged Déin Chécht that he struck his son with a sword for the third time. This time the blow penetrated the membrane of the brain but again his son was able to heal it. Unfortunately for Miach, Déin Chécht assaulted him for the fourth time and succeeded in cutting out his brain. This time he died.

Even in this legend of Miach healing himself we can see his superior skill compared to Déin Chécht, because at another time when replying to a question from Lugh asking, "what power do you wield?" Déin Chécht replied. "Any man who will be wounded there, unless his head is cut off, or the membrane of his brain or his spinal cord is severed, I will make him perfectly whole in the battle on the next day.""[2] However, when Déin Chécht strikes Miach, the latter was able to heal himself when the blow penetrated the membrane of the brain and we have seen Déin Chécht acknowledge in his reply to Lugh, that he could not heal someone if the "membrane of his brain or his spinal cord is severed." Déin Chécht's reputation as a physician was known until at least the 8th century and his charms continued to be invoked. In modern folklore, Déin Chécht's porridge is recorded as a cure for colds, sore throat, phlegm, and worms; it is made of hazel nuts, dandelion, wood sorrel, chickweed, and oatmeal.[65]

After killing Miach, Déin Chécht buried his son and subsequently three hundred and sixty-five herbs grew up through the grave corresponding to the number of his joints and sinews. His sister, Airmed, uprooted these herbs, and divided them according to their properties, spreading them out on her cloak. This annoyed Déin Chécht and he mixed up the herbs, so no one now knows their proper healing qualities.[2]

Music and chanting for healing

Chanted spells, incantations, and music were used therapeutically. Dagda's harp could play different kinds of music, which could engender sleep, joy, or sorrow, and it was not within an individual's power to resist the effects of this music.[2] The use of sound to diagnose can be seen in the following story about the illness and treatment of Teige of Mackein, a Munster Prince.[61]

---

*Elizabeth Gray, *Cath Maige Tuired: The Second Battle of Mag Tuired*. (Kildare: Irish Text Society, 1982), 52. https://celt.ucc.ie//published/T300010/index.html

Teige and Luigad- Laga were injured in battle and were carried to Tara to be cured. The physicians at Tara were induced to poison the wounds of both men, but this was to be done slowly so that there would be no suspicion fall on the King of Meath. Small reptiles, portions of poisoned arrows and an ear of barley were secretly placed in the wounds of the two men. At the same time the physicians continued to treat the men as normal as the poison was to work slowly in the background. Luigad had an argument with the king and got so exceedingly angry that his wounds burst open, and the poison was ejected. He recovered. Tadhg remained sick for a year until his own physician, Fineen, arrived from Munster with three of his most celebrated disciples.[1]

> The surgeon asked the first of the three pupils when they had heard from Tadhg a moan arising from the first wound, what was the cause of that moan. 'This is the moan caused by a prickle, as there is a barley-prickle in his wound.' On hearing a moan caused by the second wound, he asked the second pupil what was the cause of that moan? 'This is the moan caused by a live creature,' said he, 'for a live worm has been put into the second wound.' When the surgeon heard the third moan, he inquired of the third pupil what was the cause of that moan. 'This is the moan caused by a weapon-point,' said the third pupil. And when the surgeon reached the house in which Tadhg was, he placed an iron coulter in the fire until it became red hot and then got it in readiness in front of Tadhg. When Tadhg saw the red hot iron put in readiness for the purpose of thrusting it into his body, his heart trembled greatly; and, as a result of the terror that seized him, he violently ejected from his wounds the ear of barley, the worm, and the splinter of javelin-head, and thereupon the surgeon completely healed his wounds; and after that Tadhg was well without delay.

A modern-day analogy may be where an implanted metal pin or plate causes problems and needs to be removed for healing to take place.[66]

The use of song as therapy, as well as the seeming significance of the position of those seeking to help, is seen when three Ulster heroes visit

Cú Chulainn on his sickbed, where he had lain, unable to speak, for over a year. His wife, Ethne, and the three Ulster men arrange themselves at the four points around him, an arrangement we have already seen with the four physicians around the well at Slaine. Angus then sings a song to Cú Chulainn after which he is able to speak. Modern research confirms that music therapy is extremely beneficial in helping coma patients, with craniocerebral trauma, regain consciousness,[67] but the importance of the spatial position of the healer remains an area for intriguing future research.

Two other stories tell us of the physician's ability to heal psychosomatic illness. Ailill became sick with desire for his brother's wife and was taken to another dwelling to recover. He told no one what was wrong with him, and he continued to decline in health for more than a year. His brother, Eochaid, became so concerned for him that he sent his own chief physician, Fachtna, to visit him to find out the cause of his illness. He laid his hand on Ailill's chest and informed him that he suffered from either the pangs of envy or of love. Ailill refused to confirm the truth of this diagnosis so Fachtna left.[68]

The damage the pangs of envy can cause, and the power of music to heal, may be seen in the story of Covac and his brother Laery. Laery inherited the kingdom from his father and Covac became sick with envy. He found a way to kill his brother and on ascending the throne his illness left him. Not satisfied with this crime, he assassinated Laery's son also and compelled Laery's young grandson, Maon, to eat a portion of the hearts of his father and grandfather, as well as a mouse and her young. The boy was so traumatised by this experience he became dumb. Consequently, he was no longer seen as a threat by Covac and allowed leave the court. Maon moved to the south of the country, to the kingdom of Feramorc. He stayed there for some years and then went to France. While in Feramorc, Moriath, the king's daughter, fell in love with him and her passion did not decrease when he went to France. She resolved to bring him back to Ireland and to this end she wrote a love-lay, which was put to music by her father's harper, Craftiny. Craftiny travelled to the king's court in France, where Maon now resided, and played the song for him. Maon was so overcome with the beauty of the song that his speech returned to him. He subsequently returned to Ireland, killed Covac and regained his kingdom.[69]

The earliest Irish physicians

The *Genealogies of Macfirbis*[70] give us the names of the earliest physicians who came to Ireland. Capa was the first and foremost healer of his time and was all-powerful. Eaba, the female physician who accompanied the lady Ceasair, was the second doctor and she practised medicine in Ireland about 2000 BC. Slangha, the son of Partholan, was the third doctor, and Airmedh, who was the daughter of Déin Chécht, was reputed to have excelled her father in some areas. Other female physicians include Bebhinn, who practised cupping as well as general medicine, and Binn who lent her *fedan* (tubes) to Bebhinn. The Irish physicians were highly esteemed for their knowledge, and Josina, the ninth king of Scotland, came to Ireland to study medicine.

Other skills practised can be deduced from the instruments that were used. Among these were a horn called a gibne, tweezers, and a surgical probe (fraig). Cupping[+] was one of the therapies practised by Irish physicians and *Cormac's Glossary* explains the gibne or the leeche's "cupping horn" was used for this. Bebhinn, the physician, drew the venom from an old unhealed wound on Cailte's leg by means of two fedans/tubes and the leg was healed by this method.[63] There is an interesting account of Bebhinn administering five successive emetics to Cailte, who was suffering from general indisposition. They were prepared by steeping the herbs in water and each draught was different to the other and had different effects. She restored Cailte to health by these draughts, which followed the progression of the illness.

In the *Book of Leinster*[‡] there is a reference to Finghin Faithliagh, medic to Conchubhar Mac Neasa, King of Ulster in 33 AD. The king

---

[*] The Book of Genealogies was originally compiled and written in Galway between circa 1645–1666 by Dubhaltach Mac Firbisigh. Mac Firbisigh was an Irish scribe, historian and genealogist who flourished between the years 1640 until his death in 1671. The Mac Firbisigh family was a renowned learned family in late medieval Ireland. This explains his knowledge of Irish, English, Latin and Greek and his chosen 'career'. Nollaig Ó Muraíle in the introduction of his biography entitled The Celebrated Antiquary Dubhaltach Mac Fhirbhisigh (1996) states that Mac Firbisigh "represents something of a bridge between the last remnants of the native Gaelic learning classes and the new Anglo-Irish antiquaries such as Ussher and Ware." "Dubhaltach Mac Firbisigh," UCD Special collections, 08/01/2021 https://www.ucd.ie/specialcollections/archives/dubhaltachmacfirbisigh/

[†] A therapy in which heated glass cups are applied to the skin along the energy channels of the body, creating suction and believed to stimulate the flow of energy.

[‡] *The Book of Leinster* (*Lebor Laignech*) is a medieval Irish manuscript compiled circa 1160. It is now kept in Trinity College, Dublin. Previously, it was known as the *Lebor na Nuachongbála* or the *Book of Nuachongbáil*.

had been injured in battle and a missile from a sling had penetrated his brain. Finghin said that if the missile was removed the king would die. The wound was sutured successfully with gold thread to blend with the golden hair of the patient. The king was restored to health with palliative treatment but was warned to avoid all violent exercise or mental excitement in the future, as such activity could dislodge the ball and cause his death. The king got into a temper one day, started cutting down trees, and Finghin's prognosis came true. The missile was hurtled from the king's head, and he died. Another instance of the successful use of medical intervention may be seen in the story of Cennfaelad. This unfortunate man had his skull fractured during the battle of Magh Rath in 637AD. He was taken to the medical school of Tomregan where the injured portion of the skull and a portion of the brain (brain of forgetfulness), was removed. He recovered so well that he became known as Kenfaila the Learned and is credited with founding the bardic college at Derryloran in Co. Tyrone.[63]

The coming of christianity

Recorded Irish history begins in the 5th century, or possibly slightly before, with the introduction of Christianity and Latin literacy. With the advent of a written tradition, information about health and ill health can be gleaned from three main sources, namely, the hagiographical literature about the saints, *The Annals of Ireland*, and the two medico-legal law texts, *Bretha Crólige* (BC) and *Bretha Déin Chécht* (BDC). It comes as no surprise to find different approaches to illness in these sources. The hagiographical material explains illness from the perspective of Christianity, *The Annals* generally, give a natural reason for illness, and the law texts give some of the legal requirements that come into play when caring for the sick and injured.

As to be expected, there is a strong religious perspective regarding the cause of illness and the therapeutic modalities used, in the hagiographical material. The healing methods mentioned include relics, pilgrimage, prayers, rituals, blessings, and water. In religion, a relic may be described as the physical remains, or personal effects, of a saint, which are now kept as objects of reverence and a locus of veneration and honour. However, Lucas and Wycherly have shown that in early medieval Ireland relics had wider uses and that the possession of an important relic conferred considerable prestige on the owner as well as

being the means to obtain tribute.[71, 72] Furthermore, the holiness and
power associated with a relic deemed it sufficiently sacred to be used
for the sealing of treaties and the swearing of oaths. Their potency meant
they were also used as talismans in battle where, according to tradition,
they were carried in a clockwise direction around the combatants. This
clockwise movement continues today as people praying the rounds at
a holy well will still follow this sun-wise direction, as will a funeral cor-
tege on its path to the grave.

One of the most important curative belongings of a saint during
their life, and after their death as a relic, was their girdle or belt. A
story is told of a poor woman coming to Brigid* for help, but she
refused Brigid's offer of a cow or a cloak because she said they would
be robbed off her on her journey home. Brigid then gives her, her belt
because,

> you tell me there are many sick people in your part of the coun-
> try and you will heal them in the name of Jesus Christ by means
> of my girdle dipped in water and they will give you food and
> clothing.†[71]

Lucas[72] tells us that the woman made her livelihood from that day on
by curing people and the saint's injunction to give in return for healing
may possibly be seen as a precursor to giving a donation in return for
a cure, that is still evident today. An indication of the significance of a
belt for healing may also be seen in the tradition of the *brat Bríd*, which
is still associated with curative powers and takes place on the Saint's
Feast Day, February 1st.

---

*Dorothy Ann Gray tells us, the goddess Brigit, in her triadic form, represents the cor-
nerstones of Irish culture in the arts of poetry, medicine and metal work. Fire signs in the
lives of Bridget the Saint and her patronage of smithying, a craft with divine overtones,
supports her connection with a fire cult and with Irish culture.[73]

There is also the description of Brigit given by the tenth-century glossator, Cormac
mac Cuillenain and cited by Ó Catháin.

Brigit i.e. a learned woman, daughter of the Dagda. That is Brigit woman of learning
i.e. a goddess whom *fílid* (poets) worshipped. For her protecting care was very great and
very wonderful. So, they called her goddess of poets. Her sisters were Brigit woman of
healing and Brigit woman of smith-work, daughters of the Dagda from whose names
among all the Irish a goddess used to be called Brigit.[73]

†Niamh Wycherly, *The Cult of Relics in Early Medieval Ireland*. (Belgium: Brepols, 2015), 131.

The transference of the power of the saint through a relic also reso-nates with the idea of gift as developed by Mauss, where a gift always contains an attribute of the giver.[55] Part of the saint's holiness/good-ness is contained in the relic, and because of this it is able to heal. The blood or spittle of the saint was also reputed to have curative powers and this continues to the present day where the blood of certain families is said to heal shingles and the spittle of a healer "with a cure" may heal burns.[52]

Rituals, prayers, and blessings are an integral part of the therapeutic landscape and contribute to the reputation that a place of pilgrimage, a well, or even wilderness, has for restoring health and well-being, be it mental, physical, or spiritual.[73] Lough Leighis* in East Cavan was renowned for its mud, which was reputed to heal skin disease.[74] The preparation needed to participate in, and engage with, the place of heal-ing is all part of the healing process, and in early medieval Ireland local sites were by far the most popular, not least because of time constraints and difficulties in travel. It is also significant that in Ireland it is a place, be it water, hill, or stone that is the end of the pilgrim's journey, indicat-ing a perception of the land as a therapeutic entity, a place where the individual microcosm communicates with the planetary macrocosm.[75] Though ostensibly having a spiritual foundation, these sacred spaces speak of a wider understanding of healing and an acceptance of mys-tery and the inexplicable in everyday life.[76–78]

In her extensive work on pilgrimage in medieval Ireland, Nugent outlines the importance of faith and devotion in the pilgrim's hope and desire for a healing miracle in these holy places.[57] If they were healed, the pilgrim left behind proof of their malady, be it a crutch, clothing, or other talisman and quartz pebbles "have been found at several early medieval pilgrim sites."† The use of quartz stones as votive offerings left on "saint's beds" and at holy wells serve also as a reminder of how older traditions were grafted seamlessly onto Christianity as the *cloche geala*/ bright stones are associated with the *sí* and no dwelling for animal or human would be constructed with them.[79] If the *clocha geal* remind us of the Irish spirit world, then the practice of "incubation-sleeping at a holy place, in the hope of experiencing a divinely inspired dream or cure"‡

---

* *Leighis* meaning medical.
† Louise Nugent, *Stories of Faith. Stories of Pilgrimage* (Dublin: Columba, 2020), 251.
‡ Nugent, *Stories of Faith. Stories of Pilgrimage*, 254.

resonates with the incubation sleep undertaken at the Temples of Ascle-pius where people, after fasting and purification lay down to sleep, hoping that the god himself would visit and cure them during their dreams.

From hagiographical writing about the saints, as well as accounts of pilgrimage and relics, we can infer that many of the curative methods in medieval Ireland revolved around prayer, supplication, fasting, and purification. This association with holy men and women and their rel-ics, as well as the importance of holy places and holy wells, stresses the importance of the emotional and spiritual aspects of healing.[80]

More factual accounts

The Annals of Ireland speak in a different tone and are mainly factual chronicles of notable events that happened in society. They tell us about the weather, especially where this resulted in crop failure and famine causing malnutrition and starvation and the spread of disease and plague. Mac Arthur has identified the arrival of the bubonic plague in Ireland in 544–545 and the Buidhe Chonaill in 664 as well as an epidemic called the "Mortality of Children" that commenced in 683 and lasted for three years.[81] Pierce Grace,[82] in his very informative historiography of the identity of the plagues that affected the Irish population between 540AD and 795AD, notes that Wilde (1856) identified this as smallpox but McArthur (1949) categorised it as the bubonic plague. Tentative diagnoses for the major epidemics between the 6th and 8th centuries are the bubonic plague, scaly skin disorders, lameness, respiratory dis-eases, smallpox, dysentery, relapsing fevers and infectious hepatitis.[82] The Black Death arrived in Ireland in 1348 even though the Gaelic-Irish population was not as badly affected as the English inhabitants, due in part to living in more dispersed communities in the upland areas of the country. However, another outbreak in 1357 did not deal with the native Irish so kindly and they were badly affected by it.[83]

Due to the prevalence of seemingly miraculous cures rather than "any corpus of physical observations associated with scientific tests and study," Wendy Davies suggests there was little or no tradition of healing in early Irish society.[84] While alluding to the lack of written records for this period, she notes how, "the late medieval Irish texts tend to repro-duce Mediterranean material" and are "not visibly influenced by any native medical tradition."[84] Inadvertently however, Davies has identified a key component of indigenous medicine, where there may be little or no separation between the physical and the spiritual; where "art, religion and science were so closely bonded ... there were few incentives for each to prove its superiority over the others"[85] and good health was achieved through balance and harmony in one's life. Nonetheless, even though *The Annals* do not tell us about the treatment for illnesses, they are very informative because they record the many terms used for different conditions. There are six terms used for "leprosy," *sámthrosc, leprosie, clamh, clamtrusca, bolgach,* and *lobhraibh* and though this variation may refer to local idiomatic use it may also refer to differences in the presenting manifestation of the disease. *The Annals* also inform us of other terms for different conditions, such as *ficu* for haemorrhoids, *bainne aillsi* for ulcer and *aillse* for gangrene.[80]

Legal tracts

Moving to the law texts we learn about the status of the physician or *liaig*. Shaw tells us of one physician being called *suí leigis* (higher status healer) in 860, which may imply a hierarchy in the profession and a gradation of rank.[86] We have no information on the training of this physician but we do know that "a physician required public recognition before he was free to practise medicine in the tuath."[87] The *liaig* also made judgements about the seriousness of injuries received in altercations or disputes, and this assessment determined the *ériac* or fine paid to the injured party. The physician did not enjoy the same high status as the poet or brehon but was classed as a craftsman, being seen as a mechanic of the body. One legal text on distraint (the seizure of someone's property in order to pay a debt) depicts a whip and a lancet (the tool for bloodletting) as the typical identifiers of the *liaig*, thereby emphasising his role as mechanic.[42]

The legal tracts do not tell a lot about the knowledge of medicine, especially *Materia medica,* but they do tell us a little about the practice

---

*Fergus Kelly, *A Guide to Early Irish Law*, (Dublin: Dublin Institute of Advanced Studies 1988) 58.

of medicine. Binchy's examination of the *Bretha Crólige*[*] and the *Bretha Déin Chécht*[†] is comprehensive.[40, 41, 88] He informs us that both these texts relate to compensations and payments due to the physician depending on the injury sustained, or the status of a patient. There are some interesting points in relation to the surroundings for the sick person. The patient must not be asked to reside in a dwelling that he finds revolting or in a place where he feels his injury will be increased. The place must not be too bright, "where sea or waterfall or cliff dazzles…" and it must be quiet. Squealing pigs, scolding women, and the noise of children playing were all barred from the vicinity of the hospital.

In the *Bretha Déin Chécht*, (BDC) it is noted that injury to any of "the twelve doors to the soul,"demands a higher compensation. Binchy considers that, "an injury inflicted on any of them would be regarded as making considerable demands on the leech's skill and this would warrant a high payment."[‡][89] He lists them thus in his translation of the BDC:

> There are twelve doors of the soul in the human body[§]: (1) the top of the head, i.e. the crown or the suture, (2) the hollow of the occiput, (3) the hollow of the temple (temporal fossa), (4) the apple of the throat ('Adam's apple', thyroid cartilage), (5) the hollow of the breast (suprasternal fossa), i.e. the cavity of the throat, (6) the armpit (axilla), (7) the breast-bone (sternum), (8) the navel (umbilicus), (9) the … of the side, (10) the bend of the elbow (antecubital fossa), (11) the hollow of the ham (popliteal fossa), i.e. from behind, (12) the bulge of the groin (femoral triangle?), i.e. the bull-sinew, (13) the sole of the foot.

Dr Pat Logan provided him with medical reasons for each of the points.[¶]

---

[*] A legal tract mainly written by Donncadh Ua Bolgaidhi in the years 1468–74 and consisting of late translations of Latin medical works. The legal material is contained in the last 17 pages of this manuscript (No 10297 of the Phillipps MSS National Library of Ireland).
[†] *Bretha Déin Chécht* is a legal text and is also in Phillipps 10297.
[‡] Daniel A Binchy, Bretha Déin Chécht, *Ériu*, Vol. 20 (1966): 10.
[§] Binchy, *Ériu*, 20, 25.
[¶] "The equivalent anatomical terms, which are given in brackets, have been kindly supplied by Dr. Logan. To claim a fee equivalent to half of the wergild. Dr. Logan has provided me with the following medical commentary on the separate items of this list: "A severe blow on either the crown of the head (1) or the back of the neck (2) might break or dislocate the first two bones of the neck (atlas and axis), with rupture of the spinal cord.

Hindu-celtic connection

In the light of other studies in philology, law tracts, and family structure[90-92] showing Hindu-Celtic connections, a more pertinent and relevant comparison regarding the twelve doors of the soul may be formed with Ayurvedic medicine rather than biomedicine. In this medical tradition, the twelve doors of the soul appear to correspond to specific marma points.* These points are considered to be the junction points of consciousness and matter, places where the life force enters the body.[93] An injury at one of these points leads to physical and mental misery, pain, deformity, or death. Anatomically, they are points where muscles, flesh, blood vessels, nerves, bones, ligaments, and tendons all meet.

They are of specific interest in the context of compensation, as the severity of the injury can be classified according to the specific marma point affected. Firstly, are the *Sadhya Pranahara* marma points which, if injured, lead to loss of sensory and cognitive perception, as well as severe pain and immediate death. Four of the twelve doors of the soul in the *Bretha Déin Chécht*, correspond to marma points in this category. These are the top of the head (*Adipathi*), the temples (*Shankha*),[94] the sternum (could indicate the *Hridaya* or *Apastambha* point) and the navel (*Nabhi*).[95]

A blow on the temple (3) might cause rupture of the middle meningeal artery. In such a case the patient might recover consciousness quickly, and the injury would seem to be a trivial one until, some hours later, the patient went into a coma and died. A blow on the Adam's apple (4) causing a fracture of the cartilage will cause death, even now, in at least seventy- five per cent of cases. A small wound in the suprasternal fossa (5) could easily cause death from bleeding if the main blood-vessel (the aorta) or one of its branches were cut. Similarly, a wound in the axilla (6), the bend of the elbow (io), or the popliteal fossa (I1) might quickly cause death from loss of blood. An apparently slight injury in the groin (12) might also cause death from haemorrhage. A blow on the umbilicus (8) might cause sudden loss of consciousness due to paralysis of the solar plexus. The patient would recover quickly and, once more, the injury might seem a trivial one. Rupture of the bladder if it were full of urine or of the stomach might easily be overlooked at first, and these would certainly cause death. A blow in the area between the lower ribs and the crest of the illium (9) might rupture a kidney; on the right the liver might be ruptured and on the left the spleen, if this were enlarged; any of these might cause death. A blow on the breast-bone (7) might force it inwards, causing injury to the heart underneath; a twentieth-century version of this is a blow on the sternum by the steering-wheel in motor accidents | "[39] - Ériu, 20, 52

* There are one hundred and seven marma points in the body. According to Vedic wisdom, the channels of life force, called *nadis*, circulate in the human body animating and enlivening it. The marma points are where *prana* exits the *nadis* and enters the physical body. These points therefore connect the intangible prana, or lifeforce, to the physical body.

Secondly, there are the *Kalantara Pranahara* marma points and injury at these points will incur death after a period of time, usually within the month. The sole of the foot (*Talahridaya*) and the armpit (*Apalapa*) seem to fit in this group. Thirdly are the *Vaikalyakara* points, and when these points are injured, deformity results. The occiput (*Krikatika*), Adam's apple (*Manya dhamani*) Suprasternal ossa (*Nilia*), bend of the elbow (*Kurpara*), bulge of the groin (*Urvi* or *Lohitakska marma*),[96] and popliteal fossa (*Janu*) match these anatomical features. The importance of injuries at these sites may be gauged by the fact that physicians received fifty percent of the *éric* (fine) imposed, if the patient received an injury at these spots, whereas there was an increasing scale of fines based on other types of injury. For other injuries, the fines ranged from two *sets* for a *mbanbeimen* (no blemish left) to twenty-one cows for a homicide.

The story of Conchubhar Mac Neasa and his physician Finghin Faithliagh also indicates knowledge of the *Vishalyaghna* marma points. There are two such points in the body, one (*Sthapani*) is situated between the eyebrows and the other (*Utkshepa*) above the *Shanka* point (temples) along the lower limit of the hairline. The legend tells us that Finghin refused to remove the missile from the king's head because to do so would cause his death. This decision reflects the correct surgical management of this point: "The person lives as long as the *shalya* (foreign body) has not been removed. [if]The impacted *shalya* falls off by self, the person survives."[97, 98] We may also deduce that it is *utkshepa* point and not the *sthapani* (between the eyebrows) as the wound was sutured with gold thread to blend with the golden hair of the patient.

Diet and nursing care

Even though these two legal tracts concentrate on the payment due to the physician in various circumstances, they also give information on diet and nursing care. Every patient was to be fed according to the directions of the *liaig* (physician) and the basic fare was two properly baked loaves of bread every day plus different condiments depending on the rank of the patient. Unlimited celery was given to patients of every social rank due to its healing properties and garlic was also recommended. Even though garlic is deemed an estimable herb today, the Ó Cuinn manuscript of 1415[99] would disagree with this administration of garlic to everyone and tells us that it is contraindicated in people of a choleric temperament. It is interesting to note that a Moleiro facsimile of *De medicinis simplicibus* is also quite judicious in its use of garlic and differentiates between wild and domestic garlic with the former being considered more moderate.[100] There is then a difference between information gleaned from the *Bretha Cróliga* and 15th century European manuscripts. Honey is approved of in one part of the text and forbidden in another section. Salted fish or flesh were generally forbidden but not to the noble grades who were allowed it every day from New Year's Eve to the beginning of Lent and then twice a week during the summer. Fresh meat was to be given to everyone, but how often is not clarified. Boys and girls between the ages of seven and ten were entitled to the fare they would receive while in fosterage and not according to their social status. This indicates an understanding of the importance of not changing a diet, as to do so would put extra strain on the digestive system of a person already fighting illness. This text also tells us that there are three errors in nursing; the error of leaving the victim without food, the error of leaving him without the *liaig*/physician, and the error of leaving him without a substitute.[40] The latter direction indicates a well-rounded understanding of the impact of illness on a person's income and on the community.

The legal tracts, *The Annals*, and legends intimate a wide therapeutic repertoire, but detail is missing. This void is filled somewhat with the introduction of Greek/Arabic medicine from Europe, and we are introduced to that knowledge via the medical manuscripts.

Medical manuscripts

Binchy and Davies have both commented on the scarcity of literature regarding an indigenous medical tradition before 1400, and this lack is in direct contrast to the extensive corpus we have from then until 1700.[84, 101] This body of knowledge gives insight into the organisation of the medical profession, medical practices, and the medical families. Binchy tentatively suggests that this explosion in written records may be due to a need on the part of the *liaig* (physician), to display a knowledge of European medicine to maintain status. His second suggestion, in regard to the dearth of evidence regarding pre-Arabic medicine, is that Irish traditional medicine always remained an oral tradition in the older medical schools and was thus unaffected by the introduction of writing in other schools, such as those for jurists. Binchy's first suggestion is also picked up by Nic Dhonnchadha,[102] when she queries the reason why Risteard Ó Conchubhair should consider it necessary to mention that Donnchadh Óg Ó Conchubhair, who was chief physician of Ossary, had achieved his position and status without having to leave the country to study. Did this comment arise because some contemporaries were viewing a medical education obtained abroad as more advantageous for career advancement, and he was exasperated by this view? Or was it simply, that patients wanted their physicians to be educated in the Greek/Arabic medicine being taught in the universities of Montpellier, Paris, Salerno, Bologna, and Padua? This knowledge was new, and different to the traditional medicine being practised at the time, as evident in the gleanings from legend and legal tracts. As it was different to the indigenous tradition, it necessitated the translating of the textbooks being used in the European universities into Irish, so that they could be used by the students in Irish medical schools, such as Aghmacart.* The Irish medical manuscripts from this period were not simply translations, but a process that involved the editing and curating of different texts.[3] They were written in the spoken language and source texts were adapted and interpolated where necessary to suit the Irish situation.[103]

One of the medical manuscripts that were transcribed into Irish, for use in the medical schools, included translations of the *Circa Instans*.† This work has been dated to the first half of the 12th century and ascribed to Matthaeus Platearius from Salerno. It is an account of 273

---

*About a mile west of Culahill Castle the medical school of Aghmacart developed under the patronage of the Mac Giollapadraig dynasty. King James I instituted a plantation of the area of Upper Ossary in 1626 and the political turmoil affecting the Fitzpatric family at this time may account for the fact that though the school was well established by 1500 it is not heard of after 1611. This is similar to the other medical schools, some which were flourishing in the early years of the 17th century, but all of them had ceased by the 1650s (Nic Dhonnnchadha, personal communication, 2009).

†It is known as the *"Circa Instans"*, from the opening words of the text. This medieval herbal or "antidotarium" listing various herbs and their medicinal properties was compiled at Salerno about 1140–50 by one of the school's foremost teachings physicians. The family surnamed Platearius was the pre-eminent dynasty of physicians in the city during the period when the Scuola di Salerno was recognised as the leading centre for both theoretical and practical medicine in the whole of Western Europe. Matthaeus' text is a compendium of 12-century botanical science and a prototype of the modern pharmacopoeia. Copies were circulated throughout Europe, where its value was instantly recognized and where it shaped the literature of botany and pharmacy for the next 300 years."
107. Anderson, F., An Illustrated History of the Herbals 1997, Indiana: iUniverse.

herbs and minerals. Even though it deals mainly in simples,*[104] it also gives some information on their use in compound prescriptions, and their preparation.

An Irish medical manuscript that used the *Circa Instans* as its primary source, is the medical manuscript 1343 (H.3. 22) held in Trinity College Dublin. This was transcribed from Latin into Irish by an Irish *liaig*, T.Ó Cuinn, on the Feast of St Luke, the eighteenth of October 1415. This manuscript was subsequently translated into English in 1991 by Micheál Ó Conchubhair. Ó Conchubhair states in the introduction to his translation, that Twenty-three herbs mentioned in the manuscript seem to derive from a purely Irish tradition as he cannot find any reference to them in other European medical manuscripts.

Nic Dhonnchadha[43] mentions other European texts from this period, which were translated into Irish, including short passages from the Italian physician Niccolo Bertruccio (d. 1347) from Padua and Valescus de Tharanta (fl. 1382–1418) from Portugal. The *Aphorisms of Hippocrates* was translated into Irish by Aonghus Ó Callanáin and Niocól Ó hÍceadha, and their commentary on this work was transcribed many times. More than a dozen incomplete copies of their translation are extant and the earliest of these was transcribed in Lough Gara, Co. Sligo in 1413.

Bernard of Gordon was a celebrated teacher at the University of Montpellier and his interpretation of the works of Hippocrates and Avicenna influenced medical teaching for the next three centuries. His *Lilium Medicinae*,† which was completed in 1403, built upon the work of Hippocrates and the celebrated Persian physician Haly Abbas.‡ It became one of the core texts of medical teaching, as it concerned itself

---

*A simple is an account of the therapeutic effect of one herb only. It does not deal with the therapeutic effect of one herb in a compound mix of two or more herbs.

†The earliest dated extant copy of the text is in the British Library. ms Egerton 89, ff. 13ra1–192vb13.

‡Ali ibn Abbas al-Majusi (c.925–994) was known to Europeans as Ali Abbas or Haly Abbas. He is famous because of his medical encyclopaedia called *The Complete Book of the Medical Art* (in Arabic: *Kitab al-Maliki*).

This is a well-organized compendium of medical theory and practice purported to contain everything a physician needed to know for proceeding with treatment. He describes medical ethics and the importance of a healthy relationship between the physician and patients. He also refers to the use of indigenous medicinal plants, animals, and mineral products as a therapy.

with medical best practice as well as medical ethics. It was translated into Irish by Cormac Mac Duinnshléibhe (fl. c. 1459), "bachelor of medicine", and he completed it by 1482. Cormac also translated another 13th century work written by Bernard of Gordon, the *Liber pronosticorum* (1295). The *De decem ingeniis curandorum* morborum (1299), was also written by Bernard of Gordon and this was translated into Irish by Diarmaid Ó Sirideáin about whom little is known.[39]

Works from noted Arabic physicians were also translated, as well as works relating to Pharmacy[105] and surgery.[†] Arabic medicine stressed diet, environment, and lifestyle in medical treatment, and the European medical schools followed this advice. The *Regiman sanitatis* was composed by the Italian physician, Magninus of Milan, by 1334 and it was translated into Irish during the 1400s. The variety of works that were translated tell us that the Irish physicians were interested in obtaining the latest knowledge from the continent for their students and practice at home. There appears, however, to be no critical analysis of the translated works and little indication of their own native oral tradition in these translations. These works were both valued and valuable with some achieving mythical status such as the *Book of the O'Lees,* who were hereditary physicians to the O'Flahertys. This manuscript is also known as the *Book of HY-Brasil*[‡][106] because of its association with the enchanted island of Hy Brasil off the west coast of Ireland, a place where the owner of the book claimed he received supernatural knowledge of the medical cures contained within its covers.

---

*The Pharmacy tract, by Gaulterus Agilon (fl.c. 1250), entitled *De dosibus medicinarum* was translated into Irish by 1459. 108. Sheehan, S., An Irish Version of the Gaulterus de Dosibus, in Arts & Sciences. 1938, Catholic University of America: Washington DC.

†The first book of the *Chirurgia magna* (1363) of the French physician Guy de Chauliac (d. 1368) is devoted to anatomy and was translated into Irish by Cormac Mac Duinnshléibhe. Substantial portions of the lengthy *Chirurgia* of the Italian surgeon Petrus de Argellata (d. 1423), a work composed sometime between 1391 and 1423, had been translated into Irish by 1469. 46. Nic Dhonnchadha, A., Medical Writing in Irish. Irish Journal of Medical Science, 2000. 169(3): pp. 217–220.

‡RIA MS 23 P 10 (ii): Cat. No. 453 15th c. Vellum: 35cm x 25cm 92pp. The text of this manuscript is, according to A. Nic Dhonnchadha, a faithful rendering from the Latin *Tacuini aegritudinum*. 109. Nic Dhonnchadha, A., The 'Book of the O'Lees' and other medical manuscripts and astronomical tracts, in Treasures of the Royal Irish Academy Library, B. Cunningham and S. Fitzpatrick, Editors. 2009, Royal Irish Academy: Dublin.

Medical families

The pinnacle of care, education, and professionalism lay within the hereditary medical families. In Munster these families were, Ó Callanáin (Callanan), Ó hÍceadha (Hickey), Ó Leighin (Lane), Ó Nialláin (Nealon), and Ó Troighthigh (Troy). The medical families in Leinster were, Mac Caisín (Cashin), Ó Bolgaidhe (Bolger), Ó Conchubhair (O'Connor), and Ó Cuileamhain (Culhoun, Cullen). In Connaught, they were, Mac an Leagha (Mac Kinley) Mac Beatha (Mac Veigh), Ó Ceandubháin (Canavan), Ó Cearnaigh (Kearney), Ó Fearghusa (Fergus), and Ó (or Mac) Maoil Tuile (Tully, or Flood). In Ulster, the medical families were Mac (or Ó) Duinnshléibhe (Donleavy), Ó Caiside (Cassidy), and Ó Siadhail (Shields). That these medical families were proficient in their work is seen in this statement by J.B.van Helmont (1577–1644) who wrote in his *Ortus Medicinae* about medical care in the old Gaelic society.

> For I remember the chieftains of Ireland used each to give a piece of land to a healer who lived with them; not one who came back trained from the universities but one who could really make sick people well. Each such healer has a book crammed with specific remedies bequeathed to him by his forefathers. Accordingly, he who inherits the book also inherits the piece of land. The book describes the symptoms and ailments and the country remedies used for each, and the people of Ireland are cured more successfully when ill and have generally far better health then the people of Italy. (p. 13)

Ó hÍceadha (Hickey) and Ó Leighin (Lane) mean literally healer and leech, respectively. There is a well-known bonesetter by the name of Lane in the Newmarket area of Co. Cork, and it would be an interesting genealogical study to investigate if that family is descended from the old Irish medical family of the same name who resided in the Blarney area. These families were involved in the transmission of medical knowledge over many generations and as can be seen from their translations of European texts, they embraced the new learning, which was based on the works of Hippocrates, Galen, and Avicenna among others, with alacrity. The patrons of these hereditary medical families were the nobles and chieftains of Irish society. See Table I.

Table 1. The Physicians and their Patrons

Physician/Liaig	To
O'Callanan	Mac Carthys of Desmond
O'Cassidy	Maguires of Fermanagh
O'Lee	O' Flahertys of Connaught
O'Hickey	O' Briens of Thomand
	O' Kennedys of Ormond
	Mac Nemaras of Clare
O'Meara	Butlers of Ormond
O'Shiel	Mac Mahons of Oriel
	Mac Coghlans of Delvin
O'Troightig	O' Sullivan Beara

The attitude of society towards the physician is clearly seen in the status they enjoyed. Being a physician attached to one of the great Irish families was a most sought-after position, as it was well paid in land, status, and remuneration. A tract of land of up to 500 acres could have been given, and this was held free of all rent and tribute. In the case of the O'Shiels, their hereditary estate near the village of Ferbane is still known as Ballyshiel (the town of Shiel). The O'Cassidy family was another famous medical family. *The Annals of Ireland* mention the deaths of five of the O'Cassidy family, namely, Finghin (d. 1322); Gilla na nAingel (d. 1335); Tadhg (d. 1450); Feonis (d. 1504) and Feidhlimidh (d. 1520) and notes that they were *ollamh leighis* (Professors of Medicine). An Giolla Glas Ó Caiside is identified with the authorship of a medical manuscript between 1515 and 1527, which is now in the library of Corpus Christi College, Oxford.

With the Flight of the Earls in 1607, the collapse of the old Gaelic order, and the imposition of a new political order in Ireland, this medical class either went abroad or retrained, as did, for example, the hereditary physician, Owen O' Shiel.* Physicians of a lower rank may have

---

*One example of their new social situation may be seen in the career of Owen O'Shiel of the famous O'Shiel medical family. He went to Paris in 1604, three years after the battle of Kinsale. He studied medicine there but considered it "somewhat lax at and favourable in the conferring of graduation." He went to Louvain where he stayed for three years and from there to Padua where he received the degree of Doctor. He returned to Flanders

lost their profession in the new political order also, and it is possible that some of the medical knowledge of this group was disseminated into vernacular culture. The *luibh gort* (herb field), which was the main source of medicinal herbs for the ordinary people, would have also disappeared, but some of the knowledge may have remained within community lore and tradition. Threlkeld (1726) in his *Synopsis Stirpium Hibernicarum* speaks of sheaves of sea wormwood being brought from the coasts of Meath and Louth and of women selling wood sage, betony, and kidney vetch in Dublin. These are medicinal rather than culinary plants.[107]

The conclusion that may be drawn from legend, law, and text prior to 1650 is that the practice of medicine in Ireland was well organised and developed. It was overseen by hereditary families, had a wide therapeutic range, and was open to new ideas and learning from the continent. The medical families were held in high social esteem and were active in their pursuit of new knowledge. Both of these factors indicate a class who were active in their profession and diligent in the carrying out of their duties.

Herbals through the centuries

Following the demise of the Gaelic order in the early 17th century there is somewhat of a hiatus in relation to accounts about Irish indigenous medicine until the close of the 19th century.*[108] Different botanical studies were undertaken, but these were by botanists, English immigrants or

---

and was appointed chirurgeon doctor to the army of Albert and Isabella, joint sovereigns of the Low Countries. He became chief of the medical faculty in the Royal Hospital of Malines, and he worked there until 1620. In that year he returned to Ireland and settled in Dublin. He achieved fame as a doctor and was surgeon in chief of the Leinster forces under Preston. By 1646 he had transferred his services to Owen Roe O'Neill and was found among the slain between Letterkenny and Schearsaullis (Maloney, 1919). This career is very different to that of his forebears in Ballyshiel (the town of O'Sheils) who would have had a separate seat assigned to them at the royal banqueting table as well as having equal rank with the Aireach Ard (landowner). This would have entitled him to 20 retainers, 10 of whom paid him tribute. The *Liaig* enjoyed high legal status—being one of the Gaelic learned orders- in society and were supported by the hereditary tenure of lands that were granted to them by the chieftains in exchange for medical services. This was to ensure that they "...might be preserved from being disturbed by the cares and anxieties of life, and enabled to devote himself to the study and work of his profession"[108]
*The new, political order established a faculty of medicine in Trinity college, Dublin in 1711, even though medicine in some form was taught there since the early 17th century.

visiting academics.[109] Nonetheless, herbals, such as those written by Threkeld, in Dublin in 1726 and Keogh, in Mitchelstown, Co. Cork in 1736 serve as a useful record of what may have been generally available in Ireland during this time. Threkeld came to Ireland from Cumberland in 1713 and settled in Dublin, where he practised as a cleric and doctor initially, and finally settled on the latter occupation when his income improved.[109] K'Eogh was born in 1681 in Co Roscommon and after graduating from Trinity College, Dublin, was ordained into the established church. He worked as a cleric in Mitchelstown, Co. Cork. K'Eogh includes the Irish names in his herbal for a practical purpose and in his preface he advises his readers, "You will gain great Advantage by having the Name of the Herb in Irish, for in case you did not know it, or where you might find it, only repeat the name in Irish, to one of your little Botanists, and he will fetch it to you presently."[110] This decision to write the words phonetically was made deliberately,[110] so that his readers could pronounce the word correctly if they were seeking to identify it, through conversation with an Irish speaker, as he understood, "that [in Irish] so many letters have no sound at all."*,†[111] The audience for these herbals were the immigrants who had settled in the country and spoke only English. Nonetheless, both of these herbals, along with Culpeper's, are useful, because the provenance of plant knowledge today may be gleaned by examining the current use of plants by indigenous healers and tracing this backwards through these herbals to the medical manuscripts of the 15th century. This exploration of sources is also beneficial as it helps avoid a "repeated chain of ghost data" as highlighted by Renata Sõukand *et al.* in their ethnobotanical study of *Epilobium angustifolium* in Eastern Europe.[112]

This comparison helps in establishing the provenance and route of dissemination of herbal therapeutic knowledge down the centuries. Knowledge knows no boundaries and trade routes, emigration, immigration, and social intercourse have always been used to disseminate

---

*K'Eogh's orthography for Irish is apparently deliberate policy on his part. He says in his preface: "I take it to be much better to write the Irish names of the Herbs in Roman Characters, as they are pronounced, not as they are generally Spelt. For one, that does not understand to read the Irish Language (as there are a hundred to one that do not could never make Sense of them, there being so many letters that have no sound at all').

†See also, Jason Harris's discussion on the use of Latin in Irish medical manuscripts, where "Latin words are very frequently spelled in accordance with Irish phonetic laws." 114. Harris, J., Latin Learning and Irish Physicians, c 1350–c1610, in Rosa Anglica: Reassessments, L.P.Ó. Murchúhe, Editor. 2016, Irish Texts Society: London. pp. 1–25.

useful information, be it for healing or otherwise. Consequently, the following herbals were explored to help identify the possible origin of the therapeutic use of some herbs used today.

These herbals were:

1. *Medicinal Plants in Folk Tradition. An Ethnobotany of Britain & Ireland.* (Allen & Hatfield 2004)
2. *Flóra Chorca Dhuibhne.* (Uí Chonchubhair & Ó Conchúir 1995)
3. *National Folklore Schools Collection* (NFCS 1938)
4. *Luibh-Sheanchus/Irish Ethnobotany* (M. Maloney 1919)
5. *An Irish Herbal* (John Keogh 1735 [Ed] Michael Scott 1986)
6. *The First Irish Flora* (Caleb Threkeld 1735. 1988 facsimile)
7. *Culpeper's Complete Herbal* (N. Culpeper 1653)
8. *An Irish Book of Simple Medicines* (Ó Cuinn, Tadg 1415. Typescript by Micheál Ó Conchubhair 1991)

The Ó Cuinn (No. 8) manuscript serves as a valued starting point as it represents either, the Irish oral indigenous learned tradition, or the Galenic tradition as advocated at Montpellier in the 13th century. On the basis of his analysis of this text, Micheal Ó Conchubhair, the translator of the Ó Cuinn manuscript, contends that within the Irish translation there are references to twenty-three herbs that "may represent a purely Irish tradition", as there is no reference to them in any of the extensive Latin sources used by Ó Cuinn in his writing of *A Book of Irish Simple Medicines*.[99] One of the herbs included in this Irish tradition list is *Achillea millefolium* (yarrow), and by evaluating the details of this herb in the above mentioned herbals it is possible to signpost the possible origins of its current use and to ascertain if this use originates in an indigenous Gaelic tradition or the Galenic tradition. Furthermore, an appraisal of a herb such as *Arctium* sp (burdock) permits comparison with Galenic use, as this herb is identified in Ó Cuinn manuscript from 1415 as belonging to that tradition. This examination also helps us to recognise and identify the porous nature of the divide between learned and vernacular medicine.

Culpeper's herbal (No. 7) may have been popular amongst the English immigrating to this new and unknown land, called Ireland, so knowledge from this source may have circulated in the community. Maloney (No. 4) and Allen & Hatfield (No. 1) drew from certain localities mentioned within the National Folklore Schools Collection

(NFCS)* thus giving us a comparison with oral knowledge of plant use in these counties in 1938.

In the following table 2 for *Achillea millefolium* (yarrow) the learned Irish use, as outlined in Ó Cuinn (1415), is termed ILT for Irish learned tradition. The columns titled IVT represent the oral indigenous tradition in folklore and in the NFCS, subsequently written up in Maloney (1919), Uí Chonchubhair (1995) and Allen & Hatfield (2004). The columns labelled ET represent a mainly English tradition. The way 2 current healers use these herbs is also designated IVT as they are practising healers of Irish vernacular medicine today. They are designated healer B and J to protect their identity as most healers of Irish vernacular medicine are known only by 'word-of-mouth' recommendation and prefer to keep it that way. Those who have become well known, have achieved this reputation through their participation in politics, society, or sport.

Micheal Ó Conchubhair contends that *Achillea millefolium* may be a herb that represents a purely Irish tradition. The account in the Ó Cuinn manuscript is extremely brief. We are told that it is hot and dry and useful against the urinary stone and the quotidian fever. It was also used for the prognosis of a disease and in this case, three branchlets of yarrow were to be given to a patient for three days. If on the third day he vomits, he will not survive his illness, and if he does not vomit, he will survive. This brief comment illustrates the physician's confidence in the styptic and antimicrobial properties of yarrow, and the timeframe in which he expects it to succeed. If the patient vomits on the third day it indicates that the herb has not been able to staunch internal bleeding or infection and, so, will die. We are also told that it serves well against arthritis and podagra (gout), the latter linking naturally with kidney disease. Interestingly, this account also tells us that it will give a person the "gift of the gab" as long as some of this herb is kept in one's shoe when meeting someone.

Allen and Hatfield note that Pembrokeshire in Wales is the only place where using yarrow for kidney troubles is recorded, whereas there are accounts in Ireland from counties Meath and Tipperary as well as various parts of Ulster for this use.[113] In Tipperary, the root of the plant is

---

*This project was undertaken in 1938 and involved school children collecting the oral knowledge of an area. It was carried out by the senior class in every primary school in the country. This amazing collection is now digitised and available online at https://www.duchas.ie

boiled and the resulting decoction drunk, "as a cure for kidney disease"[*] but in Co. Meath, "The juice was drained off and drunk with hot milk."[†] Kidney disease could include the urinary stones mentioned in Ó Cuinn, as small kidney stones may travel down the ureter into the bladder and, if not flushed out, may grow into bladder stones.

Looking at the locations given does appear to indicate that this therapeutic application for yarrow originates in the Gaelic/Celtic tradition, even though Allen & Hatfield do not record this use in Scotland. It is also worth noting that Nollaig Ó Muraíle[114] identified quite a number of physicians of Gaelic origin in counties Tipperary and Meath in the latter half of the 16th century.

Turning to the use of yarrow for arthritis, Allen and Hatfield note that this use is predominantly Irish, and within the NFCS the frequency of this usage holds equal parity with using yarrow for divination. The general advice for rheumatism is that it should be drawn like tea and a glass taken before breakfast, but one account[115] adds whiskey to it.

> Old people got a weed called the Yarrow and washed it well. Then they cut it up, stem, leaves, roots, and all and leave it steeping for a day or two in pure spring water. Then it should be simmered for a couple of hours and strained and people add to it a glass of the best (first shot whiskey, men call it and it is not to be got in every public house) A wine glass of this mixture in water taken three times daily is a prevention as well as cure for pains.

Using yarrow for arthritis would also address the inflammatory symptoms of podagra (gout).

Turning to the third use for yarrow in Ó Cuinn, we find he recommends it for quotidian fever. This term is usually used to describe a form of intermittent malaria, but it can be used to describe any fever that recurs daily, which may be punctuated by recurrent paroxysms or cramps. It is worth noting, that despite the widespread use of this herb for fever today, this use is not mentioned in Culpeper or Threkeld. Keogh (1736), the NFCS (1938) and Uí Chonchubhair (1995) are the only accounts in the table 2 and it must be remembered that K'eogh resided in Mitchelstown. The hereditary medical family of the Ó Leighins lived

---

[*]NFCS Vol. 550: Page 274. https://www.duchas.ie/en/cbes/4922197/4860005
[†]NFCS Vol. 0699: Page 063. https://www.duchas.ie/en/cbes/5008958/4970653

Table 2. A selection of uses for Achillea millefolium (yarrow) down the centuries

Ó Cuinn 1415 ILT	Culpeper 1653 ET	Threkeld 1726 ET	Keogh 1735 ET
Use for urinary stone			
	Astringent. Reins in men and whites in women	Cooling, drying, binding. Benign gonorrhoea	Astringent. Use for dysentery and excessive menstrual flow
	Bleeding piles Restrains violent bleeding		Bleeding piles Bruise and apply to wounds to stop bleeding
Arthritis & Podagra (gout)			
Quotidian fever			Apply as a plaster with grated nutmeg on the stomach for fever
	An ointment of the leaves for all sores with moisture		
			Powdered in a glass of wine for colic
Prognosis			

IVT = Irish oral/vernacular tradition, ILT = Irish Literary Tradition, ET = English Tradition

Maloney 1919 IVT	NFCS 1938 IVT	Uí Chonchubhair 1995 IVT	Allen & Hatfield 2001 IVT	Healer B 2020 IVT	Healer J 2020 IVT
			Kidney trouble		
Powdered and used as snuff in congestive headache	Headache				
Cure for toothache	Toothache		Easing toothache		
		Arthritis			Arthritis
	Yarrow boiled in milk for a cold	Use yarrow tea for a cold		Use yarrow for colds and 'flu	Use yarrow for colds and 'flu
As snuff to draw blood from the nose			Inducing bleeding		
		As an ointment for inflamed wounds			
			Jaundice & sore eye		
	Divination	Magical purposes			

in the same general area. We may conjecture therefore, that some social interaction may have taken place between the amateur botanist and local healers and physicians.

The application of yarrow with nutmeg* as a poultice for fever, and the ingestion of powdered yarrow in wine† for cramps addresses the two issues associated with quotidian fever but this pharmaceutical detail is lost as we traverse the centuries to today, where yarrow is simply used as a tea for chills and colds. Nevertheless, there are some reports that recognise its specific action, "It is especially useful where the perspiration is obstructed a condition which is often the forerunner of fever."[116] This awareness that yarrow is used early on in a health problem is also captured in its use for inflammation. "Yarrow chopped fine boiled for ten minutes and mixed with two ounces of suet and one ounce of bees wax will cure an inflamed wound."[117] This description indicates the wound is hot and inflamed but not weeping and reflects Gerard's herbal[118] wherein yarrow is specifically referred for, "[to]close up wounds and keepe them from inflammation or fiery swelling." Using yarrow to induce bleeding appears to reflect an Irish vernacular tradition, but may be derived also from Gerard's Herbal, "The leaves being put into the nose, do cause it to bleed, and ease the pain of the migraine." This use is not mentioned in Ó Cuinn and is recorded only in Kent and Norfolk in England. This use is common in the NFCS as is the practice of chewing the leaves for toothache, a use which can again be traced to Gerard's Herbal of 1633, "Most men say that the leaves chewed, and especially green, are a remedy for the toothache." All in all, in the Irish tradition, yarrow appears to have been used as an anti-inflammatory rather than an astringent, but its applications reflect the importance of 17th century herbals in identifying how information may have disseminated among the population.

The other major use for yarrow was for divination, especially to divine who one's future husband would be. Mac Coitir[119] has identified this use in Scotland and England also even though the number of sprigs or quantity of yarrow may vary. The verse most commonly used while picking yarrow was,

> Good morrow; Good morrow ; fair yarrow
> Thrice good morrow to thee,

---

*Nutmeg is also antimicrobial.
†Wine is relaxing so will augment yarrow's antispasmodic effects.

Let me know before this time tomorrow,
Who my true love will be,
The colour of his hair,
The clothes he will wear,
The words he will speak,
When he comes to court me,

The yarrow was then placed under the pillow and while they slept, they would see their future husbands in their dreams. This divination practice was customary on May Eve or Halloween, both feasts where the boundary between this world and the other world is permeable.

Turning to the use of *Arctium* (burdock), it is probable that there is Galenic source for the use of this herb as it appears in Culpeper and Keogh as well as being in general use in Irish vernacular medicine See Table 3.

It is evident from this chart that Healer B is not isolated in his use of *Arctium* for tuberculosis (TB). It is used for TB by Ó Cuinn, Culpeper, and Keogh. Ó Cuinn uses the root of this herb on its own to stop the spitting of blood, "if the root of this herb be eaten, it will stop the spitting of blood." This indicates TB, as one of the symptoms of this disease is a chronic cough containing blood-stained mucus. Culpeper adds pine kernels to, "A dram of the roots ... [to help] them that spit foul, mattery, and bloody phlegm" and Keogh uses pineapples plus *Arctium* root for the spitting of blood.* This may be a poor transcription of Culpeper, or a synonym for pine kernels, as the availability of pineapple, or even pine kernels, in Mitchelstown in 1736 would not make this a readily available remedy for TB. Allen & Hatfield use *Arctium* for scrofula, the enlarged cervical lymph glands associated with tuberculosis, and Maloney mentions the use of *Arctium* for glandular swellings. I am inferring that he includes in this term the enlarged cervical glands present in TB. In the NFCS (1938) there are three accounts of burdock (*Arctium*) being used for coughs, colds, and bronchitis but of the fifty-one mentions therein, there is no mention of it being used for TB specifically.

Ó Cuinn says, "if the roots of this herb be boiled in wine, it will help with the urinary stones" (p. 491) and Culpeper uses the juice of the leaves of *Arctium* plus honey to provoke, "urine, and remedies the

---

*A dram of the root pounded with kernels of pineapple is a powerful remedy for the spitting of blood.

Table 3. A selection of uses for *Arctium lappa* (burdock) down the centuries

Ó Cuinn 1415 ILT	Culpeper 1653 ET	Threkeld 1726 ET	Keogh 1735 ET	Maloney 1919 IVT
TB Urinary stone Dysentery Ripening boils	TB with pine kernels	No mention	TB with pineapples	TB

IVT = Irish oral/vernacular tradition, ILT = Irish Literary Tradition, ET = English Tradition

pain of the bladder" (p. 37). K'Eogh's account is remarkably similar to Culpeper, but he leaves out the honey, "it promotes urine and breaks up the stone." From these accounts it is evident that the preparation of *Arctium* has changed from Ó Cuinn to Culpeper as the former uses wine and the latter uses the juice plus honey. In the NFCS there are six accounts of burdock being the "cure" for kidney disease, but the preparation is mainly in the form of a decoction.

Ó Cuinn uses *Arctium*/burdock also for ripening boils, "if this herb, bottom and top, be pounded and pig lard put through it, it will break and ripen boils" and there is an account in the NFCS of this use also.[120]

> Long ago to cure boils or ringworm the people used to pull the roots of a plant called Meacan Thashabha or Meacan Thashabhach. It was an herb very much like a thistle called in English the helle-bore or burdock. When it was ripe it was pulled and the roots after being washed and cleaned were put under the ashes to roast. When they were roasted, they were applied to the boil as a poultice.

This account comes from Listilleck, North, Co. Kerry and Allen & Hatfield have also identified a similar use in Co. Sligo.[121] "Boil *crádán* and poultice the boils with them." Whether these accounts apply to *Arctium lappa* is open to discussion as the Irish words used *Meacan Thashabha, Meacan Thashabhach* and *Crádán (Cnadán* also) would indicate *Arctium minus* or the lesser burdock.[119] This is highly probable as *A. lappa* is rare in the wild in Ireland, and Allen and Hatfield also

NFCS 1938 IVT	Uí Chonchubhair 1995 IVT	Allen & Hatfield 2001 IVT	Healer B 2020 IVT	Healer J 2020 IVT
Coughs, colds, bronchitis. Blood purifier. Kidney disease Skin disease Burns	Used as a medicinal herb down to recent times.	TB	TB & dropsy	Oedema

mention that different species may be involved in any discussion on *Arctium*, "*Arctium* is another example of a well-known and widely popular herb —strictly speaking herbs, for more than one species is involved ..."*[23]

Turning to dysentery, Ó Cuinn tells us "if this herb be boiled in wine, it will help with dysentery" but there is no record of this use in the vernacular tradition, either in Ireland or Britain. Using *Arctium* as a blood purifier and to alleviate skin disease is by far the most common use of this herb in Ireland and Allen and Hatfield record its use for dropsy and as a diuretic in Co. Cavan.[23] There are other unusual instances recorded in the NFCS such as *Arctium* being used to "bring out measles," alleviating the sting of a nettle, and for stomach trouble.

Any exploration of the provenance of a herb's use is therefore useful, as it shows the influence of different traditions and their diversity. It is a reminder that transmission of medical knowledge constantly occurs, but also that some factors may get lost in the process. The use of *Arctium* as currently used by indigenous healer B for TB may have come from Ó Cuinn or Culpeper (as both mention its use in treating TB), and the use of *Arctium* for dropsy from the vernacular tradition in Co. Cavan.

Healer B is an indigenous healer who manifests a sophistication, in both diagnosis and pharmacy, in his use of herbs. This advanced

---

* Allen, David & Gabrielle Hatfield. *Medicinal Plants in Folk Tradition: An Ethnobotany of Britain & Ireland.* (Cambridge: Timber Press, 2004), 280.

understanding indicates not only a careful and thorough training by his father but also the possibility that this hereditary knowledge with its many nuances and subtleties originated in a learned tradition, even though it is now oral. The understanding required to know when, or when not, to include a herb in a formula, involves knowledge of diagnosis, therapeutics, and pharmacy, all of which were taught to this healer during his long apprenticeship.

It is possible then, to trace the provenance of the therapeutic use of herbs by examining different herbals written at different times, which helps to identify the continuity of the oral tradition over the centuries to the present day.

18th — 20th centuries

The 18th to the 20th century was characterised by the growing power of professional medicine with its university graduates and "for profit" base. This paradigm was in direct contrast with the free (with the exception of donation), local, and often rural healer who was seen in their own home or local pub during a fair.[74] The other factor that addressed the emotional and spiritual health of the people during this period was the therapeutic landscape; those sacred spaces, where people could find solace, but which were also a measure of resistance to the coloniser, as well as the "native social hierarchies and priestly authorities."*[122, 123] These revered wells, hills, lakes, and woods may also be seen as a means of communion with nature, "a deeper mode of communication, more corporeal than intellectual: a sort of sensuous immersion, a communication without words."[124] The sweat house[77] was another source of healing power and energy. Foley describes them as "looking like stone igloos covered by grass and earth, the interiors were heated with turf, and patients entered and spent time in the closed settings and sweated out their fevers." †[74]

These sweat houses occur mainly in Ulster and were used in the treatment of arthritis, rheumatism, and influenza. Itinerant bath masters assessed the ability of the patient to withstand the rigours of the

---

* Ray, Celeste 2011. The sacred and the body politic at Ireland's holy wells," *International Social Science Journal*, 62 (205–206): 277.
† Foley, Ronan, "Indigenous Narratives of Health: (Re)Placing Folk Medicine within Irish Health Histories," *J. Medical Humanities* 36, 1 (2015): 8.

regime, and the presence of one of these in a small rural community provided a useful service before the advent of the all-embracing state healthcare services.

National Folklore Collection

It was recognised early in the 20th century that, due to the decline in Irish as a spoken language, the rich folk tradition present in the country would be irretrievably lost if it were not collected in a systematic manner. Consequently, in 1927 the Folklore of Ireland Society was established to save as much as possible of this rich tradition.[125] The journal of this society was titled *Béaloideas*, and its editor, Séamus Ó Duilearga, after travelling on a fact finding mission to Northern Europe, became convinced that Ireland needed "to create a national collection of folk traditions of similar proportions ... to the collections he encountered in his travels."*[125] The Irish Folklore Commission was subsequently established by the government in 1935 and since its inception has established one of the largest folklore collections in the world. The NFC, as it is now called, is held in University College Dublin (UCD) and includes, The Main Manuscript Collection, The Questionnaires associated with the collection of the material, The Schools Collection, and The Photographic Collection.†[126]

The collectors involved in gathering material for this vast project were aided, immeasurably, by a book written in 1942 by Séan Ó Súilleabháin titled *A Handbook of Irish Folklore*.[34] In this volume, the author indicates every possible type of material to be gathered, and that, "every example given throughout these pages exists as an item of tradition in this country."‡ Even though, there is only one chapter, specifically, on folk medicine,§ it is in some of the customs and practices relating to living in general, as well as the mythological and religious traditions, where we discover the attitudes and beliefs that form the envelope enclosing the remedies and cures mentioned in the chapter on folk medicine.

---

*Mícheál Briody, *The Irish Folklore Commission 1935–1970. History, Ideology, Methodology*, (Helsink: Finnish Literature Society, 2007), 19.
†Altogether, the NFC comprises over, *c*.2 million manuscript pages, *c*.500,000 index cards, *c*.12,000 hours of sound recordings, *c*.80,000 photographs, *c*.1,000 hours of video material.
‡Sean Ó Súilleabháin, *A Handbook of Irish Folklore* (London: Herbert Jenkins, 1942), ix.
§Ó Súilleabháin, *A Handbook of Irish Folklore*, 304–315.

One of the characteristics of indigenous medicine is the belief that illness may be caused by the spirit world and remaining in balance with this world is all important to the maintenance of health and well-being. Consequently, this belief informs other areas of life including the choice of a site for building a house. In 1938, Maura Fox from Co. Westmeath relates that, "You will never have luck if you build a house on a fairy path."[127] In one instance to ensure this did not happen, a priest advises a parishioner to,

> Put down ten pebbles (a yard or a foot apart) upon [the] site you have chosen in mind. You go out in the morning to check up–to see if any of the pebbles were removed. If one is missing you are not to build upon the site selected—as the house might be on a fairy path[128]

This invisible thread connecting belief in the importance and luck of certain days for house building, changing house, sowing crops, as well as healing may also be seen in the following entry:

> Many people in this district believe that if a person had cancer, he should never get a cure for it [but] only on Tuesday or Thursday. It is also thought unlucky to start house building on any day but on Monday. Nobody should change to a new house on any day but Monday because if they do, they will not live[in] it long.[129]

In like manner Margaret Cuffe from Co. Roscommon tells us:

> There are many days which are supposed to be lucky for giving cures for ailments such as heart-aches, head-aches, ring-worm, cancer and jaundice.
>
> Monday and Thursday are two days of the week which are supposed to be lucky for giving cures for heart-aches, ring-worm, and the jaundice.
>
> People do not wish to begin work such as ploughing, house building and changing from one house to another on Saturday.
>
> Friday is supposed to be a lucky day for changing from one house to another. The old saying was "Fridays flitting makes a long sitting."
>
> A cross day of the year is Saint Bridget's Day. A cross is made from straw on this day and people hand it over the door to keep away sickness.[130]

The belief in old traditions extended to cattle also.

> St Brigid founded a church in this parish at a place called Kilbride
> but only the outline of the foundations remains. Adjoining the site of
> the ancient church is a field where St Brigid, the Patroness of dairy
> farming, planted herbs for the cure of sick cattle. The late owner of
> Kilbride (Mr James Dunne RIP) who believed in the tradition, always
> grazed his sick cattle in this field with very satisfactory results.[131]

Beliefs and actions relating to the moon and healing may be seen in the
last paragraph of this account from Co. Longford.[132]

> Long ago there were more country doctors or "quacks" than we
> have at the present day. Although it was forbidden by the Church,
> it is said some people were gifted with "charms."
>   A man named Hubert Rollins living in the townland of Estate in
> the parish of Cashel has a cure for erysipelas. A swelling comes on
> a person's leg or arm. This swelling continues on for days. After a
> while, this man is called on. When he arrives, he sends a person for
> certain weeds. When the weed is got it is brought to this man. He
> takes the weed and cuts it in small pieces. He mixes these with half
> a lb. of butter. He then gets a pan and fries the mixture on the fire.
> When it is fried, he puts it on a bandage and places it on the sore.
>   It is said that if this sore is taken with new moon it will linger on
> until the moon is declining. If it is taken when the moon is declining
> it will leave when the moon is declined.[132]

These beliefs in luck, place, the moon, and tradition informed daily
actions and decisions, as well as healing and illness. This is the worldview that Séan Ó Súilleabháin is referring to when he says that many
of the cures and remedies he mentions may, "appear strange to the
modern mind, but it may be taken for granted that each had at one time
a basis which seemed normal and rational to those who used it."*[34]
    The NFCS[+] contains 8170 stories about cures and these stories vary in
their detail. They can be broadly classified into three categories, charms,

---

*Ó Súilleabháin, A Handbook of Irish Folklore, 304.
[+]Approximately 740,000 pages (288,000 pages in the pupils' original exercise books;
451,000 pages in bound volumes) of folklore and local tradition were compiled by pupils
from 5,000 primary schools in the Irish Free State between 1937 and 1939.

prayer and rituals, plant medicine, and physical manipulation. The first two will, generally, come under the term "cure" and more specifically, that such and such a person has a cure:

> There are people in Croghan that can cure diseases. Thomas Maguire cures warts. Peter Slevin cures Scurfy. Mrs Madden cures Ringworm. Thomas Mahon cures the Yellow Jaundice. John Smyth cures thorns. Michael Gilligan cures External Cancer. Patrick Piggot cures burns. Elizabeth Behon cures scalds. Mary Ryan cures the trush.[133]

Similarly, the use of blood and plants to heal may be seen in this entry:

> Mr Malach Ryan of Gregalawn cures wildfire (erysipelas). The way he cures it is he bleeds his hand or his arm three times and rubs it on the sore and says some prayers. You would have to go to him three times before it is cured. Ralph Loughnane of Kylebeg cures the measles. The way he cures them is he boils some stuff together and rubs it on them. You would have to go to him four times before they are cured. Michael Connors of Gurteen cures jaundice. The way he cures it is he boils grass and other stuff and makes a mixture. Miss Bond of Carney can cure a burn with a plaster. She makes the plaster from lard and grass and laurel leaves. She rubs it on the burn. You would only have to go to her twice before it is cured.[134]

The use of three, in this account, resonates with the perceived occult power of numbers, as well as the triskele/triple spiral so prominently displayed on the Newgrange kerbstones. Likewise, three (bleeds his arm three times) by three (visits) equals nine which is considered a significant number in many cultures for supernatural, mythical, or religious events.[135, 136] However, what is most evident in this excerpt is the

---

This collecting scheme was initiated by the Irish Folklore Commission ... [and] was originally to run from 1937 to 1938 but was extended to 1939 in specific cases. For the duration of the project, more than 50,000 schoolchildren from 5,000 schools in the 26 counties of the Irish Free State were enlisted to collect folklore in their home districts. This included oral history, topographical information, folktales and legends, riddles and proverbs, games and pastimes, trades and crafts. The children recorded this material from their parents, grandparents, and neighbours.

The scheme resulted in the creation of over half a million manuscript pages, generally referred to as *Bailiúchán na Scol* or The Schools' Collection (www.duchas.ie/en/info/cbe)

loss of knowledge. Herbs have become "grass and other stuff." Whoever is telling the boy about the cures does not appear to know that the healer collects plants with significant therapeutic properties.

There is greater detail in the following entry from Margaret Tobin, which also shows the seamless blending of visits to holy wells alongside plant cures.[137]

> A number of cures were made by quack doctors, some by charm and more with the aid of herbs. There is an herb growing in Ballintotty old castle called Marsh Mallow which cures Yellow Jaundice. This old castle is about four miles outside Nenagh. There are several cures got from "Dandeline" one which cures "Pains." Another great herb that grows is called "Cockle Root" which is great for the "Blood." They say that turf is a very good cure for asthma … the smell of the turf that is good for the sick person. Some diseases were cured by visits to holy wells at different seasons. Names of some of them are St. Conlon's well Youghal Ara. St. Patrick's well Ballywillian. St. Jacob's well Lisboney.

It is worth noting that visits to holy wells is very much part of the Irish psyche. On May 4th. 2020, during the COVID 19 outbreak, the main evening news on Irish television* had an account of people visiting and praying at St Fíonnán's well on the Iveragh peninsula in Co. Kerry. St Fíonnán was a 6th century Kerry saint and is attributed with saving people from a plague by offering people sanctuary.

More confidence in traditional cures is evident in this report, from Clooneen, Co. Roscommon,

> In this district there are a great number of cures that are handed down from generation to generation. These cures are very old and have proved successful long before iodine or any other ointment was made. Nowadays people do not try these cheap remedies and they sometimes buy in the chemist's shop things for an ailment that are not half so good as these old cures. The following is a list of these cures given to me by my mother. There were three different

*Kerry locals seek solace in holy well during pandemic. rte.ie/news/Ireland 05/04/2020 https://www.rte.ie/news/ireland/2020/0504/1136435-kerry-locals-seek-solace-in-holy-wells-during-pandemic/

cures for a wart namely, if a person with a wart saw water in a rock by accident and applied some of it to the wart after three days the wart would be cured. A snail when rubbed a wart and afterwards put on a thorn was also a cure. The snail was left on the thorn to die, and when the snail died the wart was cured. Washing soda beaten into powder and castor oil mixed together and applied to a wart was another good cure.[138]

The three cures for toothache range from the more esoteric to the more practical and efficacious.

> Teethaches were cured in three different ways. The first cure was the corpse's hand. If a person with teethaches had a near relation dead and if he or she rubbed the dead person's second finger three times along the teeth they would be completely cured but afterwards they would decay. A second cure for teethaches was to lick an "alpuker" a kind of lizard that crawls along the grass. A third cure was cayenne and whiskey. The cayenne was to be well damped with whiskey and rubbed along the teeth.[139]

The same student also recounts cures for burns and it is interesting to see the detail given about the ingredients of "garron" oil, yet the herb used in this treatment has been reduced to, "some kind of weed or slippery matter." This vague description gives the impression that this particular cure is no longer used.

> A burn was cured with cream or buttermilk. When a person was burned first the injured part was bathed in buttermilk for twenty minutes. After this, cream or garron oil was used. The garron oil was made from linseed oil and lime water. Another cure for it was some kind of weed or slippery matter that grew in a drain which was known as "loch lohan."[139]

Another cure for burns mentioned was that "The person who would lick an "alpuker"(lizard) could cure a burn" and this account comes from the same student in Clooneen, Co. Roscommon.[139] Nolan researched folk medicine in rural Ireland in the same area 50 years later, in 1989, and noted this way of acquiring a cure for burns also.[52] One of the healers he interviewed, recounted how he received this particular way of healing.*

> The cure came to him as a result of an incident which happened when he was three. He was out in the fields with his father. Some lizards (the local Gaelic word is Al Pluhar) near a wall jumped out and his father caught one and asked his son to lick it on the belly and on the back. His father then told him he had the cure for burns, and that this would remain with him until he died. Not only would he be able to cure others, but also himself. He said: "I did not feel different as a result of licking the lizard; in fact, no one knew I had done it…"
>
> He first practised his cure in the early 1940s. His father sent a local woman to see him. She had a severe scald to her right arm which was raw and made him feel sick. He described what he did then: I felt very sorry for the woman and I tried to comfort her. I made her as comfortable as I could. I then took her arm in my hands and mentally I said: 'Father, Son and Holy Ghost' and then I licked the part of her arm that was scalded. As I did so, I felt a tingling sensation in my tongue. I then sat with her for a while and after she had had a cup of tea, she went home. I saw her two weeks later and she told me that her pain had disappeared on the way home and she was now perfectly well again.[52]

More specific cures can be seen in the following entries. Mr Smyth from Kiladoon, Co. Kildare heard, thirty years previously in Co. Wicklow, that eating watercress cures rheumatism and in Co. Tipperary he heard that celery does the same.[140] Evidence of a cure being actively used may be seen in the detail given to the collector by Mrs Tate. She explains that one oz of celery seed must be boiled in one pint of water. It is then strained and drunk to alleviate the pains of rheumatism.[141]

There are over eight thousand entries for cures in general, and there are 2159 for herbs. The following entry from Co. Tipperary includes *slán lus*? (*plantego major* or broad leaved plantain) nettle, laurel and dandelion and indicates a familiarity with these cures.[142]

---

*P.W. Nolan. "Folk Medicine in Rural Ireland," *Folk Life Studies*, 27, (1989): 44–56.

The "slanless" washed and cut up cured cuts. The juice of a dock leaf was put to peeling lips; a dock leaf also cured nettle rash. The root of the dandelion steeped in sour milk cured warts, the stem of dandelion was a cure for teeth aches. The laurel leaf was boiled in lard and reduced to pulp; the mixture was applied to burns to cure them. Robin-run-the-hedge (*Galium aparine*) was boiled and drank as a cure for chest trouble.

There are also accounts which include the treatment of other animals.[143]

The names of the weeds that are growing around here are lamb's-quarter, rag-weed, chick-weed, thistle, dandelion, yarra, garlic, broom, bulkyshans, heiferans, scutch, browns-wort, feather-few, nettles and wild celery ... The dandelion grows very plentifully in this district. If it is boiled down and if the juice is drunk it will cure rheumatism and all pains in the feet. It will cure boils and pimples off the skin. It is often chopped up and mixed with a handful of meal and given to pigs to eat. The leaves are often given to rabbits in a cage to eat ... Garlic is good for the black leg in cattle.

Yet other accounts cover herbs used as simples.

A fistful of oatmeal was added to a bucket of spring water to allay thirst. which is a very practical use of oatmeal.[144] Water on its own resolves thirst, but the addition of oatmeal, because it has a low glycemic index, assuages hunger. This means work can continue for longer before breaking for a meal.

The practical use of herbs can also be seen in the use of oak bark to prevent the harness chafing a horse's breast while working.[145] Oak bark was also used to prevent foot soreness in cattle. The informant, Michael Rooney, gives a significant detail in his account; it is the bark off an old oak tree that is used. The bark must be boiled before bathing their feet in it, and as the lotion dries on the skin, a protective coat is formed that hardens the skin and prevents chafing.

"Butcher's broom" or *Ruscus aculeatus* was boiled for blood pressure, but whether it was high or low blood pressue that was being treated is not stated. Modern research supports the use of broom for orthostatic hypotension,[146] so these accounts may be referring to low blood pressure. Nettles seem to have been the more popular herb for this condition, "nettles are a cure for blood-pressure, and they are also a blood purifier and a tonic,"[147] but leeches and blood letting are also recommended, "To cure blood pressure a patient must put a leech on his chest, which sucks the blood,"[148] and "The remedy for High Blood Pressure was blooding letting."[149] There is an account from Bannow, Co. Wexford, which says that broom was also used for dropsy (congestive heart failure), "Gilteac or broom, as it is sometimes [called], boiled and the water drunk is a cure for Dropsy."[150] Another account from Co. Mayo tells us that, "People pull broom, and boil it, and when it cools, they put sugar init(sic). When this is done, they drink the juice, and this is generally said to be a good cure for dropsy."[151] *Cytisus scoparius*, also known as broom top, is a potent diuretic; and diuresis is needed to relieve pressure on the heart in congestive heart failure.

Willow (*Salix sp.*) or sally rods were used in different ways and show how versatile people were in their use of a plant. Externally, sally rods plus calico were used by the bonesetter for binding fractures.[152] They were considered effective since they are firm but supple. Willow bark (sally rods) contains salicylic acid, which is both anti-inflammatory and analgesic. This anti-inflammatory effect of willow is also evident in a treatment for erysipelas, a skin infection. In this case, the sally rods are burnt and the ash mixed with herbs and some thick cream. This paste is applied with a feather, and three *Paternosters*, *Aves* and *Glorias* are said. This procedure is repeated three times, Monday, Thursday and again the following Monday.[153]

There are vestiges in this account of the need for connecting with the supernatural and a recognition that healing comes from the spirit world. Lyons reports that a Lillooet shaman used a feather for divination purposes and that eagle feathers were also used as rain medicine objects,[154] while Eliade in his seminal work on shamanism gives many examples of the use of feathers in shamanic costume and ritual.[155]

The cause of vitamin deficiencies may not have been known, but the correct choice of a plant to treat the symptoms is evident in the use of brooklime. A collector for the National Folklore Commission (NFC), P. J. Ó Suilleabháin, reports that the herb brooklime (*Veronica Becca Bunga*)* was chewed and applied to sore lips in Lispole, Co. Kerry.† The cause of the sore lips is not stated, but traditionally brooklime was

---

*National Folklore Collection (NFC) Volume 752 ends at page 310 and the entire volume deals with clothes and dress. The data relating to NFC 752: 363 is taken from the index cards only.
†National Folklore Collection. Volume 752: Page 363 index card only.

pounded and applied to sores such as bleeding mucus membranes (gums and lips), which are a sign of scurvy. Allen and Hatfield record the use of brooklime in Counties Cork and Kerry, where it was used for colds and coughs as well as for the symptoms of scurvy.[23] Brooklime has abundant Vitamin C, which makes it very useful in both conditions, as modern research shows that vitamin C boosts the immune system thus helping prevent further complications in respiratory complaints. Brooklime was also used as a diuretic, to treat kidney and urinary troubles and as a spring tonic.[23]

A plant may be utilised in different ways in different counties as can be seen with the elder (*Sambucus nigra*). The green part of the elder forms the ingredient of a traditional remedy for sores*[156] in Kerry and in the same county, Lispole, the bark is used in a formula that was made up as an ointment for burns.[†] The inner part of the bark is green, so both accounts could be using the same part of the tree. The elder leaf was used for treating a varicose ulcer in Co. Wexford, the informant, J. Maher, is quite detailed in his description:[157] the leaf is held in front of a fire until the juice begins to leave it; once this occurs the inferior side of the leaf is placed on the ulcer. Mr. Maher informed the collector that he cured several people with this single herb. Again, the knowledge and use here is very much cause and effect and appears to have been acquired through observation and use.

There are some unusual cures evident in the NFC, such as the account in NFC volume 1838, pages 175–176 where a remedy for diabetes involves immersing a young frog in spring water and then swallowing it. It is a cure so foreign to our sensibilities that our rational mind dismisses it as a *piseog*; but we could be wrong. Current research is showing that several frog skin peptides stimulate insulin release and show promise as a treatment for patients with type two diabetes.[158]

Indigenous medicine is often understood as a folk variation of scientific medicine and is seen through the lens of scientific medicine using the same conceptual tools.[9–11] But examining indigenous/folk medicine from the viewpoint of scientific medicine is inadequate because indigenous/folk medicine needs to be explored as part of a cognitive system wherein health care reflects a people's philosophy and cultural tenets.[9,13] Donna Maria Wing in her comparison of the concepts implicit

---

*NFC. 744:10
†Data taken from index cards, plant category.

in traditional healing and modern healing explains this very succinctly, when she tells us that within folk cultures, "healing and spirituality are one", whereas Western biomedicine separates out the "body from the mind and the soul."*[159] This insight, as well as the blending of different spiritual traditions, is evident in this account from Co. Kilkenny in 1938.[160]

There is only one holy well in the parish of Galmoy. It is Saint Bede's and the townland of Bayswell is called after it. The well is coffin-shaped and none of the old people remember any cures to happen there.

There are two Holy Wells in my neighbouring parish where many cures were obtained in olden times. One of them is in the townland of Fertagh, which is only a short distance from where I live. It is called *Tobair na Ciarain* and there are many stories told about the well. When Saint Kiaran was at Fertagh, he sent his maid for water to the well. He noticed she was staying a long time. When she did not return, he went to look for her. He found human bones from which the flesh had been lately torn by some wild beast. He gathered the bones together, and he prayed over them. In a few moments he discovered his own maid. The big flag where this miracle was performed is still to be seen at the well.

The other holy well is on the border of the parish, and it is called *Tobair na Suil* or the well of the eyes. In olden times, many people from all over the country and outside countries visited it and many cures are reported to have taken place in it. There is a little bush growing in the well and people who visited it placed ribbons on the bush as mementoes. Many years ago, a farmer living near the well would not believe it was blessed. He went one day for a bucket of water to boil turnips. He placed a great fire under it, but he could not get the water to boil or if he had it down until now it would not boil. He believed in the holy well ever after when he saw this.

Even though the National Folklore Schools Collection was undertaken in 1938, this blending of healing with cultural views remains strong today. Moore, in his study of attitudes to the "cure" in Northern Ireland,

------

*D.M.Wing. A Comparison of Traditional Folk Healing Concepts with Contemporary Healing Concepts *Journal of Community Health Nursing* 15 no 3 (1998):145.

observed that people are very comfortable moving between traditional and modern methods of treatment, especially if old ways are deemed to work well.[161] This efficacy is evident in the following three accounts, which were utilised within the last thirty years.

The first account is about a woman whose son had whooping cough. The boy was two and a half and despite the many cough bottles that were prescribed repeatedly by the GP, there was no improvement in his condition. A parent from the school rang this lady and told her she had a cure for whooping cough. It consisted of alternate layers of swede turnip* and brown sugar in a bowl. The bowl was then covered with a tea cloth and left for twelve hours. As soon as the mother returned home from work, she layered half a suede turnip with brown sugar and covered the bowl. At nine pm she heard her son go into a paroxysm of coughing and decided to give him the liquid that had gathered in the bowl without waiting for another six hours. The coughing stopped and he slept the night. The cough went entirely in a few days.

The following two cures have natural causes *i.e.*, ringworm, and a sprained ankle, but tthe method of healing is beyond current medical understanding.

Two young boys had contacted ringworm from playing with kittens and there were hundreds of spots all over their bodies. Their mother obtained a prescription from her GP, which was a cream. She had to apply this to each of the spots three times a day and she was no sooner finished with one child, when she would have to start on the other. This continued for most of the summer until one day her mother-in-law suggested that she take the children to a neighbour who was the seventh daughter of a seventh daughter. The boys' mother was sceptical about the powers of the seventh daughter of a seventh daughter to cure ringworm, but she took the children to her anyhow. This woman, who was in her seventies, "very very lovingly laid her hand on each of the spots" and the woman was most impressed with her caring attitude. There was total quietness while this activity was being carried out. The boys' mother stopped using the cream and within two to three days the spots began to fade. That cure was effected about twenty-three years ago in the early 1990s. It took place in Ballinamore, Co. Galway.

---

*Swede turnips, or *rutabaga*, differ from the smaller white turnip or *Brassica rapa*. The former are commonly called swedes in Ireland.

This cure took place in Limerick city many years ago where a certain gentleman had a jewellery shop. One of his employees, Mary, sprained her ankle but still came into work. It was very painful and very swollen. Her employer suggested that she return home, but she refused. He then arranged her work so that she could remain sitting inside the counter. A protestant clergyman came in to get his watch repaired and, while the jeweller was doing this, the clergyman started talking to Mary. Her sprained ankle became the subject of conversation and the clergyman said that he "could deal with that" for her. He asked her to come outside the counter and sit on a chair. She duly did this and was very mystified. He knelt down on the floor, took her ankle between his hands and said, "sit there quietly while I say a prayer." The prayer took about one minute, even less. The jeweller could not hear it as it was said *sotto voce*. The clergyman then stood up and said, "Now dear, in about an hour that will be fine." He finished his business in the shop and left. Mary returned to her work and by the time she went home two hours later, the swelling in her ankle was gone, she was able to walk on it and it was completley better. Her employer considered the whole event very mysterious but said "it happened, and I saw it happen."

Going to see a healer with a "cure" is in itself an acknowledgement that there is more to healing than visiting a medical doctor and reflects the "mortar binding a distinct and fundamental value system."[*][161] It also requires effort as most healers do not advertise, and knowledge of them belongs to the "word-of-mouth" domain. The majority are unknown outside the localities in which they operate, and for Nolan this dislike of public exposure may be deemed part of the "quack's ... unwritten code of practice" where "they never advertise their services ... they never declare openly that they have a cure, nor do they speak about those who possess other types of cure."[†][52]

This reticence to speak openly about vernacular medicine is a change from the 19th century where writers such as Lady Wilde and Lady Gregory had no problem with recounting tales of healers such as Biddy

---

[*] Ronnie Moore, "A General Practice, A Country Practice: The Cure, the Charm and Informal Healing in Northern Ireland" in *Folk Healing and Health Care Practices in Britain and Ireland*, 104–129, edited by Ronnie Moore and Stuart Mc Clean, (Oxford, Berghahn Books, 2010).
[†] Nolan, "Folk Medicine in Rural Ireland," 45.

Early*, as well as illnesses caused by the "Good People", such as the changeling, the fairy blast and the evil eye. So, what were the events that brought about such a decisive sea change in worldview that, even though the cure is still part of the cultural paradigm, it is becoming increasingly marginalised and only spoken about if asked?

---

*Biddy Early was a healer in Co. Clare who was renowned for her healing abilities. She was deemed to have received her gift of healing from the fairies. Roman Catholic priests were particularly hostile to her activities and discouraged people from visiting her.

CHAPTER 3

Change and decline

A changing worldview

Within indigenous societies, the world of invisible or spirit entities is part of the worldview and their presence influences daily living. This feature is present in Irish folklore. In the preface to *Ancient Legends of Ireland*, Lady Wilde affirms the Irish respect for the invisible world, and the strange and mystical superstitions associated with it.[29] She says that this belief in unseen spirits, "even in the present time, affect all the modes of thinking and acting in the daily life of the people" and is ubiquitous in 19th century Irish rural life.*

> Every act of the peasant's life has always been connected with the belief in unseen spiritual agencies. The people live in an atmosphere of the supernatural, and nothing would induce them to slight an ancient form or break through a traditional usage.

Sean Ó Suílleabháin refers to this belief in the fairies differently. He refers to it as a reality "for our ancestors."[34] This belief in the existence

---

*Speranza Wilde, *Ancient Legends, Mystic Charms, and Superstitions of Ireland* (London: Ward and Downey, 1888, 1971 edition) 188.

of the fairies may be seen in many areas of life, even to the siting of a
house, because building over a fairy path could affect the occupants of
the house by bringing bad luck. The respect shown to the fairies can be
seen in accounts of food being left out for them, and in the offerings of
poteen or milk poured on the ground for their use.[162] Lady Gregory
mentions that, "They are everywhere;"*[33]

This belief in an invisible otherworld influencing daily life is also seen
in medicine. Ó Súilleabháin noted that people were more impressed by
the "ceremonial curing of a complaint, by the recitation of an often corrupt
spell or charm (ortha), as well as by complicated acts and gestures", than
"the straightforward cure of an ailment by the application of a plaster."[163]

But, if the practices of daily life change because the old ways are
no longer functional, then the worldview changes also. Ó Súilleabháin
was able to say that the customs, beliefs, and patterns of life associated
with daily life were, "highly practical measures, deeply concerned with
human life and welfare. Far from being casually evolved, they were
in the main serious attempts to protect vital human interest and were
relied upon by the folk in times of crisis or danger, whether fancied
or real."[163] Similarly, Glassie, in his exploration of life and living in
Ballynemone, reiterates the point about the practical nature of customs
and beliefs, and their role in addressing the many questions about life
and the world in general, when he tells us that, "Things must be useful. Bridges, songs, houses, tools, land—like food and tales and good
neighbours—should help carry you on."[164] Thus, the stories, customs,
work methods, and rituals evolved in society, sustained the daily work-
load, the sorrows, and the joys in a community. But when an object or
custom was no longer useful, it was adapted or discarded. When the
old worldview no longer meets the needs of daily life it evolves and
changes. This change is seen in Mrs Day's sons no longer believing in
the stories about the fairies, and even more telling is a reply Lady Gregory received from a person she had asked about his brother's visions:[33]

> If it was a young man told us of them we might believe him, but as
> to him, we pay no attention to what he says at all. Those things are
> passed away, and you—I beg your pardon for using that word-a
> person—hears no more of them.†

---

*Augusta Gregory, Visions & Beliefs in the West of Ireland (Buckinghamshire, Colin Smyth
Ltd, 1920, 1970 edition) 9.
†Gregory, Visions & Beliefs in the West of Ireland, 203.

CHANGE AND DECLINE   75

Gregory's *Visions & Beliefs in the West of Ireland* captures a changing social order in relation to healing and these accounts are worth examining as they help to illustrate the disruption of the Irish indigenous worldview after the famine in the 1840s. The change in relation to healing is apparent in the following stories.[33] Mrs. Nelly of Knockmogue, tells the following tale:

> There was a girl lived there near the gate got sick. After waiting a long time and she [was] getting no better the mother brought in a woman that lived in the bog beyond, that used to do cures. And when she saw the girl, she knew what it was, and that she had been overlooked. And she said, did you meet three men on the road one day, and didn't one of them, a dark one, speak to you and give no blessing? And she said that was so. And she would have done a cure on her, but we had a very good priest at that time, Father Hayden, a curate, and he used to take a drop of liquor and so he had the courage to do cures. And he said this was a business for him, and he cured her, and the mother gave him money for it. It was by herbs that women used to do cures, and whatever power she got in the gathering of them, she was able to tell what would happen. But she was in great danger all her life from gathering of the herbs, for they [the fairies] don't like anyone to be cured that they have put a touch on.

Fr. Hayden can cure, she says, because he takes a drop of liquor, and his fear of the fairies is thus dissipated. His ability to cure is in contrast to an account that is given elsewhere by Wilde, where the mother of an "overlooked" child calls the priest for help but he refuses because he was afraid of the fairies.*

In these two accounts, we see that the knowledge and power of the *bean leighis* gradually yield to that of the priest. The priest is consciously taking the task away from the woman with the herb cures, "And he said this was a business for him." He does not cure with herbs, so that knowledge, and "whatever power she got in the gathering of them" disappears as peoples' need for her disappears. The preternatural world is being moved aside, as well as the knowledge needed to

---

*All that night the child cried and would not sleep. And all next day it moaned as if in pain. So, the mother told the priest, but he would do nothing for fear of the fairies.[32]

Wilde, S., Ancient Legends, Mystic Charms, and Superstitions of Ireland. (1971 ed.). 1971 ed. 1888, London: Ward & Downey, 21.

communicate with it. There is a financial transaction also, "the mother gave him money for it", which is in direct contrast to that reported by Wilde about the fairy doctor.[29]

> The fairy doctor must pronounce from which of these three causes the patient is suffering. The fairy stroke, or the Fairy Blast or the evil eye; but he must take no money for the opinion given. He is paid in some other way; by free, gracious offerings in gratitude for help given (p. 232)

The mother in the instance quoted above is seen to be moving between two worlds. She brings in a woman from the margins, "a woman that lived in the bog beyond", to find out what was wrong; so she trusts this woman to diagnose. She then dismisses her (even though "she would have done a cure on her") in favour of the priest who was a good priest, because he drank and, "had the courage to do cures."

This shift of the power to heal the evil eye from the *bean leighis* is evident in other tales also. Mrs Clerey speaks about her two sons who were cursed by a woman.[33]

> And they pined a long time. And I brought the one that was so bad over to Kilronan to the priest and he read over him. It was a lump in his mouth he had, that you could hardly put down a spoonful of milk, and there was a good doctor there and he sliced it, and he got well. But the priest often told me that but for what he did for him he would never have got well. (p. 82)

In this instance, it is clear it is the modern medicine that cures the young man. The woman with herbal cures or charms does not enter the picture at all, and the priest who reads prayers is also ineffectual. However, the priest continues to remind the mother that only for him the boy would not have got well. The role of the priest in this instance (and others) is very similar to traditional healing for mental disorders in Saudi Arabia. This healing often consists of reading verses from the Holy Koran to the patient, but does not involve the use or ingestion of herbal substances.[165] The tension between the old and the new may also be reflected in the family where the mother did not go for help for her son, "I never went to anyone, or any witchcraft, for my husband wouldn't let me but left it to the will of God; and anyway at the end of the eleven months he died.'"[33] In this vignette, the old ways have become witchcraft; the lack of responsibility in seeking help appears to have been reduced to a fatalistic submission to the will of God.

These narratives also indicate that the clergy have become the new healers of the effects of the evil eye. However, the use of this power appears to bring consequential loss. Fr. Mulhall lost his milch cow, and Fr. Gardiner his horse. Fr. Heseltine lost his health, and when a priest in Ennis did a cure it broke his heart.[†][33] There is no intimation from the accounts recorded by Wilde that anything untoward happened to the fairy doctors, but we are told by a Mrs Manning‡ that both priests and Biddy Early could suffer loss.[33]

> A priest has the power to do cures, but if he does, he can keep nothing, one thing will die after another … Biddy Early could do the same thing, she had to cast the sickness on some other thing—it might be a dog or a goat or a bird.

This consequential loss intimates at a position analogous to what Mgbeoji[13] says about sacrifice. He says events that upset the equilibrium between the supernatural world and the human world include natural disasters, epidemics, and violation of societal norms. These infractions indicate that the balance between both worlds needs to be restored and "restoring the social and cosmological equilibrium may take the form of several types of sacrifice and other means of rearranging social and cosmological order."[13] In the narratives discussed here, the individual has no choice; the *sí* do not like their intended victim escaping, and they inflict hardship in some other way. This misfortune is evident in a number of accounts told by Lady Gregory, of which the following is one example.[33]

In this instance a woman is extremely ill after having a child and her husband sends for Fr. Rivers, who said, "Which would you rather lose—the wife or the child—for one must go? The next day the baby died and so did a "fine cow out in the field, but the woman recovered and is living still." There is an implication in this story also that Fr. Rivers moves between the clerical world and the Otherworld because he dies

---

*Gregory, *Visions & Beliefs in the West of Ireland* 93.
†Gregory, *Visions & Beliefs in the West of Ireland* 96–98.
‡Gregory, *Visions & Beliefs in the West of Ireland* 99.

within two years. The reason given for his premature death was, "They never live long when they do these cures, because that they say prayers that ought not to say"[33] (p. 98).

This passing of the baton from the healer to the priest, is evident from the narratives recorded by Wilde in the 1880s, through those recorded by Gregory in the 1910s, and on to the NFC from the 1930s onwards. Over this period, the narratives suggest that the use of divination, rituals, herbs, and incantations by the wise woman/man has been superseded by the clergy using their invocations and prayers.

This change in a society's perception of their world may occur for many reasons. This may be sharp and violent in the case of genocide, or gradual in the case of colonisation. In the latter case, adaptation to the new political order develops after the initial turmoil of conquest, and the subjugation of the indigenous worldview and knowledge is more gradual, but no less effective.[6, 15] Seán Ó Súilleabháin, in *Irish Folk Custom and Belief*, intimates at such a displacement when he says that folklore changes continuously, but slowly due to an innate conservatism. He explains this slow change to the fact that the customs, beliefs, and pattern of life among a rural population, will not change unless there is a major change in society such as that brought about by, "famine, plague, war, invasion, colonization or mass migration."[166]

Famine: the great hunger

A "major change," displacement, or disruption occurred in Ireland during and after the potato famine of the 1840s. The rural poor were the ones who suffered most; it resulted in mass emigration in the latter half of the 19th century and the first half of the 20th century. In 1870 there were 1.8 million Irish in the United States who had been born in Ireland.[167] Emigration led to a decline in traditional values, as the emigrants had to adapt to new work practices, a new society, and for many of them, a new language. Emigration thus created an awareness among the emigrants, and those who stayed at home, that traditional beliefs may not help in the achievement of worthwhile goals and may no longer be useful in a new and changed society.[15]

A national system of primary education

Even though there were various attempts at providing education before 1831, that year marked the introduction of a national system of primary education. This meant social advancement through education was achievable, but, unfortunately, the medium of learning was English. Consequently, many parents encouraged their children to speak only English at all times, as did the government and Church.[15, 168] This adoption of English as the spoken tongue by the younger generation in Ireland may have resulted in the loss of plant and therapeutic knowledge between the generations, as well as the values associated with them. Knowledge of indigenous medicine is most commonly transmitted from mother to daughter, with many of these plants included in family meals.[169] Ó Tuathaigh, referring to the fatalism that accompanied the language shift from Irish to English, suggests that it, "clearly influenced the language that they wished their children to speak,"* and in an end note (No. 48) comments that, "The issue of gender in the language-shift—specifically, the influences of mothers on their children within the home—awaits close investigation."[168] That shift in language also signposted what the people perceived to be more useful and valuable, as well as having more status. This issue of status may still be evident, and can be seen in this account, where a younger lady (age, mid-thirties) was admonished by her aunt (age, mid-sixties) for sending her two children to a *Gaelscoil*, which is a school where the medium of teaching is Irish.†[170] The conversation ended with the aunt saying, "Only the poor speak Irish." This exchange illustrates a disapproving attitude towards Irish as a native tongue, and it is an attitude that has passed down through the generations among sections of the population. It is a view that is still prevalent, because speaking Irish is not perceived to be advantageous in progressing through life, and was/is associated with demoralisation, poverty, and backwardness.[4] What is perhaps even more significant in the loss of language is David Abram's theory that a people's language, how it sounds, how it flows, is an expression of the land in which it evolves. This point of Abram's is most eloquently illuminated in Manchán Magan's, *Thirty Two Words for Field*, a lyrical paean to the details, nuances and subtleties in the Irish language and a reminder of a different worldview.[171] To stop speaking a language is therefore a detachment from the land, and the underlying beliefs and practices which are an expression of the relationship between people, language and land.[172]

---

* Gearóid ÓTuathaigh, *I mBéal an Bháis* (Cork: Cork University Press, 2015) 32.
† A. M. Keaveney. Conversation with author, Dublin, 2011.

This attitude pertains specifically to the Irish language and does not identify other customs, traditions, and practices of an indigenous Irish worldview which may also have been affected by such negativity, including indigenous medical practices. Adopting a form of medical care associated with the established middle class may also have been deemed progress, and one exchange helps to illustrate this. A herbalist suggested a particular plant to a patient for her presenting condition, and the patient remembered using this plant as a young woman. She remarked how she stopped using it once they were able to pay to visit the doctor, as the neighbours then knew they had "come up in the world."

The Roman Catholic Church

Another factor that may have contributed to the displacement of Irish folk medicine was the rise in power and influence of the Roman Catholic Church after the famine. Three aspects of this rise in power and influence are germane to the exploration of the decline in Irish indigenous medical practices. There are many stories relating to the opposition of the clergy to the "wise" woman/man, Biddy Early, "The priests were against her and used to be taking the cloaks and the baskets from the country people to keep them back from going to her."(p. 37)[33] In the latter half of the 19th century, the Roman Catholic Church was able to be more active against the wise women, and the fairy doctor, since the number of priests, monks, and nuns ministering to the Catholic population had increased steadily from 1800 to 1850 and even more rapidly between then and 1900. Larkin[5] in his discussion of the "Church, State, and Nation in Modern Ireland" cites McCarthy's[173] comparison of the clerical population to the Catholic population in Ireland during the 19th century.

> In 1800 there were about 1850 priests, including some twenty-six bishops, in Ireland for a Catholic population estimated at 3,900,000, or roughly a ratio of one priest to 2,100 faithful. There were also in 1800 only 122 nuns in Ireland, which if reduced to a ratio divides out at the meaningless proportion of one nun to 32, 000 ... In 1861 there were 5,955 priests, monks, and nuns for a Catholic population of 4,505,265; in 1901 there were 14,145 clergy for a population of 3,308,661 ... or a ratio increase from 1: 1000 in 1850 to 1: 235 in 1900.

Secondly, in the area of education, there was a successful devolution of power from the Establishment to the Roman Catholic Church in this period. In 1878 when Archbishop Cullen died, "the education that existed for Catholics in Ireland was largely controlled by the Church," and with the establishment of the National University of Ireland in 1908 this control of education extended, unofficially, to university. Thirdly, Larkin, in his analysis of the Roman Catholic Church and its role in the rise of the modern Irish state, argues that the adoption of a more Roman Catholic lifestyle, including regular Mass attendance, was brought about by a collective identity crisis. This crisis was caused, "by the increasing loss of the Irish language, culture and way of life during the preceding century."[174] He argues that the church gave the people a substitute symbolic language and offered them a new Christian cultural heritage with which they could identify, and by which they could be identified.

Larkin also recognises that a more Roman Catholic lifestyle was adopted in the latter half of the 19th century. The embracing of this lifestyle may be measured by the increase in attendance at weekly mass from thirty-three percent before the famine to over ninety percent within fifty years. He ascribes this uptake to the collapse of the whole peasant belief system,[5] which was the popular religion in pre-famine Ireland and which co-existed with the official and canonical system that was the Roman Catholic Church. This popular religion comprised celebrations, magical observances, and superstitions and was tied to the agrarian year. The main celebration was the harvest, and when the harvest failed during the famine years of 1845–1848 the credibility of this popular system collapsed, thus paving the way for the triumph of the canonical system.

Economic progress

It was the "respectable" and economically better off Catholics who practised their religion before the famine, and this group were left relatively unscathed by that awful decade. The potato failures of the 1840s and the resulting starvation, disease, and emigration, affected the cottiers, paupers, labourers, and landless much more than these devotional adherents, so this class benefitted the church with an even more solid core after the famine than it had before those tumultuous years.[175]

The values and mores of the Roman Catholic Church complemented the economic needs of the farmer after the famine. As a percentage of the population, farmers who had thirty acres or more before the potato failure increased from seven percent (7%) in 1841 to nearly thirty two percent (31.9%) in 1901. This growth contrasts with the decline in farm holdings between one and five acres. These decreased from almost fifty percent (44.9%) of all farm holding in 1841 to slightly over twelve percent (12.2%) in 1901. (P. 877)[174] Thus, farmers in general wished to maintain the economic gains achieved over the preceding decades and their hunger for land continued, because the movement from tillage to grazing necessitated larger holdings. Between 1850 and 1878 this wealthier, better educated and Catholic community emerged, but their new-found security was threatened by three harvest failures in 1877, 1878 and 1879 as well as the Long Depression in farming between 1873 and 1896. The possibility of eviction and emigration spurred this class into political activity and the Land League was formed in 1879. The main aim of this movement was to get rid of landlordism and the purchase of farms by the tenants. Many Roman Catholic clergy participated in the Land League and this support, plus political manoeuvrings, resulted in different land acts between 1883 and the Wyndham Land Purchase Act of 1903. This latter act set the requirements for breaking up large estates and allowed for the transfer of ownership of land to tenants. This success further fastened the identification of Roman Catholicism with an Irish nationalism that valued economic progress and a new modern worldview, so aptly described by Ó Súilleabháin in 1967, when speaking about Irish indigenous medicine.[163]

> Folk belief, in the sense of superstition, was bound to be at variance with modern cultural outlooks, and has been opposed through public education, as well as through religious teaching and other means, not excluding ridicule. (p. 12)

Added to this, was the development of formal medical structures where professional medical bodies "created an identifiable group of trained professionals for whom the practices of folk medicine seemed anathema." (p. 8)[74] These formal medical structures also meant a hierarchical structure of formal medical training in established universities, and a denigration of the indigenous practitioner who had learnt as an apprentice. It was a power struggle and the medical establishment won.

Social hegemony

The question then is, why was indigenous medicine not included in the great Gaelic revival of Irish culture that took place in the latter half of the 19th century and early part of the 20th? In 1893, Douglas Hyde, who became the first President of Ireland, established, with Eugene O'Growney and Eoin Mac Neill, the Gaelic League to protect and encourage the preservation of Irish culture, its language, music, and dance. This led to the publication of many books on Irish folklore, the establishment of the Abbey Theatre and a flourishing of Irish art, drama, and literature. As well as the resurgence in the arts and literature, indigenous Irish sports were revived, and thrived, under the auspices of the Gaelic Athletic Association (GAA), which had been founded in 1884 with the aim of establishing an organisation to renew and nurture traditional Irish sports.

In a speech to the National Literary Society in Dublin on November 25th, 1892, Douglas Hyde stressed the necessity for de-anglicising Ireland because he wanted to show,

> the folly of neglecting what is Irish, and hastening to adopt, pell-mell, and indiscriminately, everything that is English, simply because it is English ... this failure of the Irish people in recent times has been largely brought about by the race diverging during this century from the right path, and ceasing to be Irish without becoming English ... with the bulk of the people this change took place quite recently, much more recently than most people imagine, and is, in fact, still going on.[176]

Hyde and his contemporaries were more than successful in their efforts to bring about a revival in the arts and literature, but nowhere is there a mention of the indigenous cures, the plants, the rituals, the charms.

The reason for this may lie in two areas. The first is function. Many writers, Glassie, Ó Súilleabháin, Moore and McLean, among them, stress the importance of something having to be useful if it is to survive. "Things must be useful. Bridges, songs, houses, tools, land—like food and tales and good neighbours—should help carry you on."[164] Similarly, Moore tells us, that among the people he interviewed, the old cures continued to be used if they were effective. Farmers still use cobwebs when dehorning cattle because it works, but there is no longer a need to hang a cloth in the dairy to develop mould to treat pneumonia because antibiotics are available.

The second possible reason why indigenous medicine was not developed is that the establishment of free primary education allowed families to become upwardly mobile, to move in polite social circles, and adopt the manners and mores of the Victorian middle class. Literacy had improved considerably by 1901, with only slightly over sixteen percent considered illiterate, whereas there were nearly forty-six percent considered so in 1861.[175] Likewise, the sons and daughters of farmers who had achieved relative economic security in the latter half of the 19th century, and early 20th century could now enter the professions of law and medicine, as well as the church, since the National University of Ireland had been established in 1908. Why this social class, in any country, would hasten, "to adopt, pell-mell, and indiscriminately, everything that is English, simply because it is English" has been discussed by Kwasi Konadu in his exploration of indigenous medicine in Ghana.[6] He says this adoption of values other than their own comes about, because a people who are colonised will only value what the coloniser values, and they learn, during the centuries of oppression, to despise the aspects of their own culture that were not valued, enjoyed, and appreciated by their political masters. The Anglo Irish exalted, encouraged, and patronised Irish music and literature, and were instrumental in the establishment and flowering of the Gaelic revival. This aspect of being Irish was therefore valued. This point of Konadu may be further illustrated by the furore on January 26th, 1907, the opening night of John Millington Synge's play, *The Playboy of the Western World* in the Abbey Theatre. Riots broke out as nationalists considered the play to be an insult to public morals and Irish womanhood rather than portraying the Irish as a sober, self-reliant people. In other words, it did not depict the Victorian milieu the newly arrived bourgeoisie wished to emulate and portray.

Indigenous medicine with its "cures" and "bottles," charms and rituals would not fit into this world where a different medical paradigm prevailed. By incorporating the Western medical paradigm into their worldview, the Irish middle class were simply doing what the hereditary medical families had done centuries before when they brought back to Irish medical schools the Galenic medical tradition from Salerno and Montpellier. The difference this time was, rather than integrating the new with the old, the indigenous tradition was actively discouraged, and this may have been because the worldview had moved from cyclical to linear, holistic to rational, pattern to cause.[177]

Nevertheless, there were attempts to introduce accounts of Irish indigenous medicine to a wider audience, the most distinguished probably being the short account, *Medicine in Ancient Erin*, published by Burroughs Wellcome for the British Medical Association meeting in Belfast in 1909.[108] In 1919, a small book entitled *Luibh-Sheanchus/Irish Ethno-Botany and the Evolution of Medicine in Ireland* sought to, "give in outline the evolution of Medicine in Ireland and to indicate the comprehensive character of Irish Ethno-Botany" with the author in the preface reproaching England's pedagogy for the lack of knowledge of Ireland's nature creeds.[178] The author, Michael Maloney, stresses that, "from the economic point of view alone Irish folk botany is worthy of attention" and,

> at all events it is not too much to hope that a study of the Ethno-Botany of the Celts allied with the Pharmacology of today may win back some of the fame of the Irish physicians of the long ago and help at the same time the common cause of humanity. (p. 9)

There were other nascent attempts to establish a herb-growing industry in the country, but they did not succeed. In 1919 Christina Quinlan, a lecturer in botany in University College Cork, published a pamphlet on how to wildcraft herbs. This was published by the Commissioners of National Education in consultation with the Irish Herb Association.* Its aim was to stimulate an interest in wild plants, not only as a science subject but, "as a means towards the establishment of an Irish industry of considerable value at all times."[179] Among the herbs to be wildcrafted were coltsfoot, celandine, dandelion, sloe, bilberry, buckbean, henbane, broom, yarrow, comfrey, fox-glove, couch-grass, agrimony, mullein, elder, burdock, centaury, meadow saffron, male fern, and wild valerian.

In 1933, Tadg Foley's *Medicinal and Perfumery Plants and Herbs in Ireland*[180] was published and, here again, the author hoped that a herb growing industry would be established. He mentions, in particular, the profusion of *Artemesia maritima* growing wild in Galway Bay and the Shannon Estuary where, in his opinion, it could be harvested for

---

*The Irish Herb Association had four branches, Leinster, Ulster, Munster and Connaught.

its medicinal value. He mentions the establishment of experimental plantations but only mentions two locations, both hotel gardens. These experimental plantations may be the ones referred to by O'Reilly in his paper on "Essential Oils and Medicinal Herbs" published in *Studies* in 1933, where he says, "semi-technical scale plantings and distillations … yield essential oils of a character equal to the best Mitcham oils and perfumes."[181] Joseph O'Reilly was Professor of Chemistry at University College Cork and he urged the establishment and development of an industry based on essential oil extraction from herbs, especially lavender, peppermint, and dill. It can be observed from these efforts to establish an industry based on herb production that the approach to indigenous medicine was economic, and nowhere is the other arm of this medical paradigm mentioned, namely, charms, prayers, and rituals. Neither is there any exploration of this indigenous knowledge as a medical paradigm. The plants are being seen from a pharmaceutical and economic perspective only.

CHAPTER 4

Utilising Irish indigenous medicine today

It is evident that the changes which have occurred in Irish society in the last century have had an enormous effect on our perception of Irish indigenous medicine. It is not possible for us to revert to a worldview that sees the "good people" in a swirl of dust, but, just as the currach changed from a boat used for fishing to one for pleasure, so can the riches of indigenous medicine be used to enhance our health today. This is possible because our worldview is again changing. We have become more conscious of the earth as a fragile ecosystem, a home we have to nourish, and care for, rather than coerce and exploit. Our survival as a species depends on how we interact with the planet, and this involves the development of a holistic approach to life in general. Frenetic activity is not good for health or spirit.

By following the rituals of the Irish calendar year* a more reflective, sustaining, and nourishing lifestyle can be engendered. This lifestyle can incorporate the different qualities that are essential to our complete health, namely, the emotional, spiritual, rational, and physical attributes

---

*The Irish calendar year refers to the key times (and corresponding festivals) in the agricultural year, such as planting crops, moving cattle onto grass after the winter, harvesting, etc.

of our being, all of which are present within Irish indigenous medicine and the Irish calendar year.

From the day we are born, to the day we die, we respond to our environment with our feelings, be it fear, joy, anger, or distress. Each day gives ample opportunity to allow the processing of these emotions, and our ability to do this will determine our emotional health. Suppressing emotions is not healthy, nor is allowing them free rein the answer. Taking due cognizance of our emotions, without being overcome by them, indicates an emotionally healthy person, one who is self-aware, has strong coping and adaptive skills, and is able to manage stress. The obverse is a person unable to express their emotions in an appropriate manner, repression, lack of self-care and the possibility of severe anxiety and depression.

The spiritual side to living is, all too often, seen as the domain of religion when it is in fact rooted most often in our experience of nature. The natural landscape is not inert and man's response to it is often expressed in spiritual terms.[77, 182] By learning to listen to nature, to observe and be quiet in its presence, we open the core of our being to the primal source of Tao/Being that emanates from every atom of the universe. This sense of wellbeing and peace is supported by research in Japan, where an increase in natural killer cells, and a reduction in stress hormones, has been noted when people visit forests on a regular basis.[183]

In Ireland, the divine is often sought in liminal places, numinous locations where, "the presiding spirit of the place becomes an intercessor with the ultimate divine, rather than being divine."(p. 271)[123] This sacred landscape includes water, stone, and wood, and examples include Croagh Patrick and Lough Derg, as well as the numerous holy wells scattered throughout the country. Pilgrimages to these places are not visits to a church to see a saint's relic, but journeys to locations where the sacred has been experienced for thousands of years. These are settings, where the early Christian missionaries, "syncretically folded pagan places of pilgrimage, including holy wells and sacred trees (bilí), into the new faith,"(p. 271) managing to retain, integrate, and harmonise both forms in the process.[56]

Our reason and intellect are developed by learning. Whether one is nine or ninety it is important to be always open to new thinking, new knowledge, new ideas. This not only keeps our brains alert but allows us to integrate the old with the new, and to pass this wisdom to the next generation. To be always learning allows us to become elders, honoured for wisdom, esteemed for discernment, loved for caring.

Physical health is deemed necessary by everyone, and it is achieved by exercise. Physical exercise may be more difficult for some people due to underlying physical problems, but no matter how little, it is vital to our health.

The Irish calendar year is based on the cyclical nature of agriculture, which creates an awareness of the cycle of food production on which we are all dependent. Introducing aspects of Irish vernacular medicine which are evident in this calendar allows us to incorporate the different pillars of healing into our lives. We reach back through the centuries, not only to prehistory, but to the wider community of Western Europe from which so many Irish people originated. By utilizing the local traditions of healing, we link also to the wider world such as the United States of America where so many Irish people emigrated and where vestiges of Irish indigenous medicine still exist in Appalachian folk medicine.[184] Adapting and incorporating the rituals associated with the significant seasons of the Irish calendar year is a walk through tradition, where each year something extra can be added, so that over time there is a seamless integration with the cyclical year and its unfolding.

Spring

Imbolc/St. Brigid

Even though the Irish calendar year commences at *Samhain*, on November 1st, it is more appropriate for us to start our journey in the Spring, with the feast of *Imbolc* on February 1st which is also St Brigid's Day. *Imbolc*, along with *Samhain* and *Bealtaine*, is celebrated within the family unit and was celebrated well into the second half of the 20th century. Some of the rituals associated with this feast are easily updated to create a welcome break during the cold, and often bleak, weather after Christmas. St. Brigid along with St Patrick and St. Columcille form a triad of Irish saints who have lived on in Irish consciousness. Despite centuries of devotion, her historicity is inconclusive, and she may well represent and incorporate the accomplishments of, "several early Christian women, as well as those of indigenous Goddesses and Mary, the Jewish mother of Christ."*[185]

Imbolc was originally a pagan festival, and can be translated as "ewe-milk," "parturition," "heavily pregnant," "suckling" or, literally,

---

*Maeve Brigid Callan. "The Safest City of Refuge": Brigid the Bishop. Gender, Sanctity, and Power in Medieval Ireland." In *Sacred Sisters*. (Amsterdam: Amsterdam University Press, 2020) 87.

"in the belly," thus reflecting the burgeoning fertility at this time of year. Cows are in calf, ewes in lamb, and mares in foal. The days are visibly lengthening and even though the weather may be appalling the first signs of new growth are beginning to emerge. This is the day when everybody involved in food production can begin to plan for the year ahead. By dedicating February 1st to ordering seeds, deciding on garden crops for the year ahead, and assessing the remedial work needed on window boxes, planters, garden beds, and allotments, we are connecting with tradition and the communities of old. By assigning this task to *Imbolc*/St. Brigid's Day also gives food production the honour it deserves, and prevents it being the hurried endeavour it often is, come March and April.

In days of yore, especially, in Kerry and West Cork, no one would undertake work that required the turning of a wheel at this time. This tradition can be renewed today by becoming a day for walking only; no cycling, no car, no train, simply a day to travel at a slow pace and enjoy one's surroundings, be it the architecture of the city, a local parkland, the dunes by the sea, or the paths on a mountain. By its very nature, this activity is local and gives the opportunity to chat with neighbours, notice the immediate environment, and observe the changes that have taken place over the winter. It also reminds us that walking is the most basic and valuable of humans' means of transport. The sights and sounds of the day, the impressions and musings, the conversations and insights may be noted in a log or E portfolio entitled *Imbolc*. Over the years, such a record will provide valuable information for the next generation as well as triggering memories of days gone by.

In Irish cosmology the day starts the evening before with night being a time of preparation for the day ahead. This belief has its roots in observation of the natural cycle as all life begins in darkness, be it the seed beneath the soil, the chick in the egg, or the baby in the womb. For that reason, the celebratory meal in honour of St. Brigid takes place on the eve of her feast day and the traditional fare included colcannon, barm brack, apple cake, and dumplings. Butter always formed part of the meal and the meat served was generally mutton or bacon. To continue this tradition acknowledges that we are links in a chain, and it is our task to teach the next generation how important each link is. We are not self-sufficient, and decisions made today by individuals and societies may strengthen that chain or break it entirely. The serving of traditional food may, then, serve as a starting point for a discussion on the necessity of good food for health, but also to a conversation about the food chain, logistics, and local suppliers. Vegetarians and vegans have the opportunity to adapt the traditional fare, and colcannon is a firm favourite since it is simply cooked cabbage mashed into potatoes and served with butter. Different foods may be served in different localities, with pancakes being served at Brigid's supper on the eve of *Imbolc* in Ulster.[186]

St. Brigid was believed to travel the country on this night, blessing each household, people, and livestock as she passed by. It was customary to place a slice of cake, or bread and butter, on the windowsill to welcome her, and a sheaf of corn for her "favourite white cow which accompanied her on her rounds."*[187] In a custom reminiscent of *Samhain*, an extra symbolic place was laid at the table for the saint, and the food was later given to the first poor person who came begging. Today, this tradition can translate into donating to a food bank or to famine relief charities.

The most widespread custom associated with February 1st is the making of the St Brigid Cross from rushes, (See images 1 and 2) and the making of these crosses continues in many a rural school today. There are local variations but the most well-known is the one with four arms. The oldest type of cross in Ulster had only three legs, and this was hung in the barn to aid fertility in the animals, whereas the crosses with four legs were blessed in the church and afterwards hung in the house to protect it from harm, especially fire and lightening.[188]

The tradition of making crosses is one that can be continued today and, as before, hanging the cross above, or on, the entrance door can be accompanied by some ceremony, such as lighting the candle on Christmas Eve. Danaher tells us that in some parts of the country the cross was blessed with holy water, and its hanging was accompanied by the following prayer; "May the blessing of God, Father, Son and Holy Spirit be on this cross and on the place where it hangs and on everyone who looks at it."†[187] This prayer can be adapted to the spiritual beliefs of the household, but what any invocation acknowledges is that the unexpected can happen, and the need for protection and security is a constant in our lives.

---

*Kevin Danaher, *The Year in Ireland* (Cork: Mercier Press, 1972) 15.
†Danaher, *The Year in Ireland*, 19.

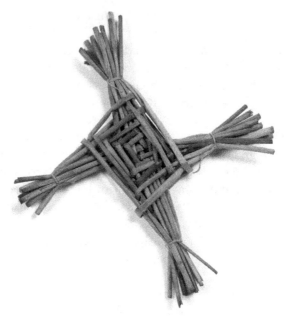

'Four-armed cross of rushes from Clonfert, Co. Cork. © National Museum of Ireland.'

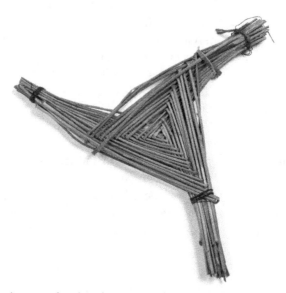

'Three-armed cross of rushes from Cruach Leac, Co. Donegal. © National Museum of Ireland.'

As mentioned previously, Brigid gave her girdle to a woman, so she could earn her living by healing, and the tradition of the *brat Bríd* continues that connection with compassion, generosity, and healing. The custom today involves a piece of cloth being left outside for Brigid to bless as she passes by. This is then kept for the year and is believed to have curative powers. It was considered especially effective against headaches, tooth ache, and earache.

Sacred wells are to be found across the globe because, "... water symbolises the whole of potentiality ... the source of all possible existence."[*][189] Another tradition associated with St Brigid is to visit one of the many wells dedicated to her. People then brought home some of the water and sprinkled it on the house, its occupants, and farm buildings. It would be an interesting exercise today to locate any such wells in one's local vicinity and visit them. Seeing how water bubbles up from beneath the ground to renew the earth is a lesson never forgotten and taking some of the water home to bless the house is an acknowledgement of the absolute essential nature of water in our daily lives.

St Brigid was always seen as protector of the heart of the house, yet she is also associated with liminality, between worlds, neither in nor out. She is reputed to have been born on the threshold of the dairy, her mother having one leg inside the door and one leg outside. It is also said that she was born at the breaking of the dawn and her red-eared white cow links her with the world of the *Sí*. Accounts of her life in the *Vita Prima* and *Bethu Brigte*, portray a world in which pagan and Christian freely intermingled, yet she is extolled as a Christian saint; a woman who bridges the gap between heaven and earth.[185] Her hospitality was immeasurable, and she was readily able "to turn water into milk or beer depending on her guests' needs."[†][185] She was so in harmony with nature that she was able to hang her cloak on a sunbeam and all nature was subject to her.[‡]

This ability of Brigid to stand between worlds can serve us well today as we reflect on choices we have to make, and understand perhaps, that the old does not always have to be discarded but can, instead, be integrated with the new. A household is a unit in itself, but its members

---

[*]Eliade, *Patterns in Comparative Religion*, 188.
[†]Callan, *Sacred Sisters*, 94.
[‡]Callan, *Sacred Sisters*, 110.

are also part of a wider community as soon as they cross the threshold. Brigid is a reminder that we all have to live and make our choices in that liminal space between private and public, self and other, past and future.

Imbolc/Brigid's Day is, then, a rich source of emotional, spiritual, physical, and intellectual sustenance. If Imbolc/Brigid's Day falls in the middle of the week, and it is not possible to observe it on the day, it is possible to turn the weekend after it, or before, into a family festival to celebrate this patron of the Irish.

This celebration is achieved through:

- Not turning a wheel and walking only
- Having a celebratory meal and laying a symbolic extra place
- Making St. Brigid's cross
- Planning the garden for the year ahead
- Donating to a food bank/charity
- Discussing the world of food and what is needed to maintain it
- Locating and visiting a well dedicated to St Brigid
- Reflecting on the nature of liminality and its meaning in our lives.

St Brigid's flower

The dandelion is known as St Brigid's flower and is a very useful herb. The young leaves may be used in salads, and to reduce some of the bitterness in the leaves, blanch them by placing a pot over some plants for a few days. Brigid was famous for the home brewed ale she served all her visitors, so Imbolc may be an opportune time to make some dandelion wine from the young dandelion crop. In 1938, Maureen O' Conner gave this recipe for making dandelion wine,[190] but there are many more available today.

> People make dandelion wine for cures. Gather two quarts* of dandelion petals, boil, stir, and cover with a flannel cloth and leave for three days stirring now and again. Then strain them. Put the water into a pan and boil for half an hour, with the rind of lemon, and a little ginger. Then slice the lemon into it and add one and a half pounds of sugar. When cool put in a bit of bread with a quarter

---

*One quart = 37 oz or 946 g.

ounce of yeast and leave for two days; Then put in a jar and leave for a day or two.

Dandelion leaves are diuretic and for this reason a tea made from them increases urination so may help in urinary tract infections.

Dandelion tea is made as follows:

Pick four or five leaves and wash quickly. Chop or tear into pieces. Place in a small ceramic/china teapot and pour water, that is just coming up to boil, over them. Put the lid on the pot and let infuse for 10 minutes. Strain and drink.

St Patrick's day

Six weeks after celebrating Brigid, Ireland enters festive mode again in honour of Patrick. Even though this festival is now celebrated across the globe Danaher tells us that there are only two practices that derive from tradition, and these are the wearing of an emblem and "drowning" the shamrock.[187]

Wearing the shamrock, or a cross, has been recorded in Ireland as early as 1681 and Dean Swift mentions the Irish wearing crosses on the Mall in London on St Patrick's Day in 1713.[191] Similarly, in 1766, "his Excellency Count Mahony, Ambassador from Spain to the court of Vienna, gave grand entertainment in honour of St Patrick" and all those present, "to show their respect to the Irish nation, wore crosses in honour of the day, as did the whole court."(p. 59)[192] Today, the wearing of the cross has died out and has, generally, been replaced by a harp with a ribbon attached or by pinning a posey of shamrock to one's coat lapel. To celebrate this day, collecting the shamrock could become a foraging expedition in addition to being a test in identifying it. A bowl of shamrock could grace the dinner table, and this does not have to be as elegant as the one usually pesented to the US President, but instead, a reminder of all our families and friends who are part of the Irish diaspora.

It is also a good day to retrieve the family tree, and note those who had to emigrate and why. These stories can form part of the family history to be passed down through the generations and could be recorded using a voice recorder and/or written down. It is a day to honour our forebears who struggled and survived to allow us to live in better times.

St Patrick's Day normally falls in Lent and the *Pota Pádraig/* St. Patrick's pot denotes the drink taken on this day, but also the term used for any treats given to children, since having a drink or eating sweets is a relief from the traditional abstinence associated with Lent. Drowning the shamrock does not mean drinking to excess, but the tradition of placing the shamrock that had been worn during the day, into the final glass of punch and a toast then being made. Once that was over, "the shamrock should be picked out from the bottom of the glass and thrown over the left shoulder."(p. 65)[187] This tradition is one that could be easily adapted to a celebratory meal at home with a toast raised to absent family and friends.

St Patrick, Brigid of Kildare, and Columcille are considered the major triad of Irish saints, yet we have no feast day to Columcille, and Brigid's Day is almost forgotton. A home school project, or family discussion, could involve why this has happened, as well as exploring the stories of Brigid and Columcille to identify aspects of their lives that are relevant to us today. The storyteller in the family could also entertain with an account of the lives of one or more of this triad. Storytelling is a therapeutic goldmine, as the listener is able to resonate with a different part of the story at different times. The story of Columcille tells of pilgrimage or exile, the significance of a safe place, and being honoured in another country rather than in Ireland. Exile, sanctuary, and making a success abroad, are as relevant today as in the 6th century.

St Patrick's Day can, then, be a family festival that enriches our sense of belonging to the countryside, and to our history. This is achieved by,

- Searching for shamrock
- Wearing shamrock
- Making a table centrepiece of shamrock
- Attending a parade
- Exploring the family tree
- Discovering why family or friends now live abroad
- Making a toast to absent friends and family
- Contacting friends and family through social media
- Exploring the stories of the triad of Irish saints, Patrick, Brigid of Kildare, and Columcille for their relevance today.

Easter

The next major feast in Spring is that of Easter, which, because of public holidays in Ireland, is always a four day break. As Easter can occur anytime between March 22nd and April 25th, it is a fitting occasion to examine the role of the moon in time-keeping and the significance of the Spring equinox. The tradition of Easter is determined as being the first Sunday after the first pascal full moon after the vernal equinox[*] and it was decided upon in 325 CE at the council of Nicaea. Easter is a more than fitting time to examine how man manages both the solar and lunar movement of our planet. It is also the time to examine the different celebrations that occur at the vernal equinox throughout the world. This activity reminds us that the passage of the earth around the sun determines so much of our lives and our food production. Again, it reinforces our connection with the earth, and the universe.

We are so used to calendars that we forget they are man-made. How would we measure time if we did not have one? It is easy to forget that standardised time zones were not estabished until the late 19th century, and only then because of the need for uniform times for train travel. Prior to that, local time applied, and one had variation, obviously, from city to city. The Greenwich meridian is the prime meridian today for time zones, and Easter is a perfect time to establish solar time for where one lives, as well as establishing the solar orientation of the home. Exploring the difference between the solar and lunar calendars is another activity, and one could also investigate why the night sky would be important for the Inuit of Canda to find their way.

Another activity for gardeners is to explore the biodynamic system of cultivation, as it uses the waxing and waning times of the moon for planting and harvesting. This new information may identify some test plots to determine if there is sense in this method of growing vegeatbles.

The east-west orientation of the passage tombs at Knowth suggest an equinox alignment, but a better example is at Loughcrew, Co. Meath. This was built to align with the spring and autumn equinoxes so it would be an enjoyable early morning excursion for those living near it, or those who have come to Ireland to celebrate St. Patrick's Day. Further afield is Grianán of Aileach, which dates from 1700 BC and is situated on a hilltop in Inisowen Co. Donegal. This stone fort is associated with Dagda, a god of the Tuatha de Danann, who is reputed to have ordered it to be built as a monument to his son who had been killed. Any trip to

---

[*]The ecclesiastical vernal equinox is set as March 21st. The vernal equinox can vary, however, between March 19th and 21st.

a site of a local neolithic monument to determine its alignment would link us to these early settlers and how they used stone to determine the journey of the earth around the sun. Such a foray to the countryside can also involve exploring the history and geography of an area to find wells, rivers, rock art, and old monuments. Photographs can be taken and recorded in a video or scrap book to peruse during the winter months, or even added to one's Christmas greetings to show the return of the sun and another growing season.

Traditionally, Good Friday was a time for visiting the graves of one's forebears and this is an important ritual for a family. It teaches the continuity of life and respect for the ancestors. Like Ash Wednesday, it teaches the fragility and transient nature of human life. Emotional health is bolstered by honouring one's ancestors. This can be lighting a candle, recalling anecdotes about them, and visiting their final resting place if that is possible. Photographs of the different styles of graves and gravestones evident in any graveyard can lead to seeking the answer as to why this is so. A visit to a grave may result in an entry in a diary where one reflects on the impact ones' parents, grandparents etc. have had on your life, be it positive or negative. If negative, it may be time to ask if one's life is still affected, and if so, what steps need to be taken to resolve it and move on. It may involve the realisation that contact with grandparents is important for children, as it links them to so much knowledge about family and history as well as transmitting skills and information.

There is a lovely tradition throughout Ireland of people going to hilltops on Easter Sunday morning, as the rising sun was supposed to dance with joy at the resurrection of Jesus. It is a tradition worth keeping as it is a message of hope, the realisation that after darkness there is always light. One could say that light is always present in the dark just as dark is the inbuilt aspect of light. We know, always, that one will turn to the other just as day follows night. If Easter day was fine, many holy wells were visited, especially if they were known locally as Sunday's well. Long walks in the countryside were also undertaken.

Easter is a family time, when the new fecundity of the earth is reflected in the chocolate easter egg, but there are many traditions associated with eggs at Easter that may be usefully initiated if suitable to a family or community. These include painting and decorating eggs, and in some districts, hitherto, these were kept to decorate the May bush at *Bealtaine*. Danaher tells us that in many parts of the north of Ireland, hard boiled eggs were rolled down a hill and if one egg smashed into that belonging to another, then the owner of the uncracked egg won both.[187]

The Simnel cake, though more an English tradition, is very popular in Ireland and its rich ingredients of nuts and dried fruit are nutritious as well as tasty. The decoration of eleven almond paste "apostles" pays homage to it being a vehicle as a moral story, telling of the betrayal of Jesus by Judas and how he lost his place among the apostles as a result. Such a visual impact of loss of status can be re-interpreted to include the importance of loyalty, but also, at what point does one have to say, "I have to follow my own path."

Easter, because of the lengthening day, also sees the beginning of outdoor activities and an outdoor dance was commonly held on Easter Sunday. This would have occurred in the evening, and would have been an opportunity to discuss and meet others from the neighbour-hood and further afield. Today, it can still involve a community celebra-tion or media communication with family and friends.

Easter then gives an opportuntiy to,

- Discover the various festivals worldwide associated with the spring equinox
- Examine the importance of the solar and lunar calendars to food production
- Explore antiquities in your vicinity
- Visit a graveyard and ponder on the architecture therein as well as praying for those who have died
- Update the family tree and individual histories
- Bake a Simnel cake
- Decorate eggs and start an egg rolling competition
- Have a family celebration.

Valuable food and plants in spring

In days of yore, the health of the family was considered part of the mother's domain, and to this end she gathered herbs to make into teas, juices, syrups, wines, and creams. The plants associated with spring are dandelion, chickweed, plantain, and sweet violet. I have already dis-cussed how dandelions may be added to salads, as well as made into wine, but the others are just as useful.

Chickweed/*Stellaria media/Fliodh*

This herb was used for swollen joints, and this use has been recorded as early as the 15th century, as well as in the records of the NFCS. In the 15th century it was boiled in water, pressed well and pig lard and butter added to it. This was then placed as a plaster on the affected part whereby the pain was reduced. Today, the pig lard and butter could be replaced by beeswax and oil, with care being taken to whip it well while it sets; otherwise, it will become too hard and the water element will fall to the bottom. Keep refrigerated and use for strains and sprains when required.

Plantain/*Plantago major/Slán lus*

Even though Plantain is seen by most people as a nuisance its virtues are too numerous to mention. The NFCS records its use for healing cuts, but one account says the smooth side draws a boil while it is the rough side heals a cut. Another description says to chew it before applying to the cut, but this was not common. Br. Angelo Mac Shámhais received this information from P. Mac Shámhais:[193]

> *Slánlus* is the handy application for all kinds of cuts. The clean leaf is pressed into the gushing blood where it soon sticks fast. It is not removed until the wound heals. (I have seen a quack chewing the leaf and applying the pulp to the bleeding wound. B.A.)

Allen and Hatfield[23] record other uses for this herb, such as plantain juice for a cough and applying the leaves for burns, as well as drinking the boiled juice for liver trouble and jaundice.* What is interesting about these uses is that they are also recorded in the Ó Cuinn manuscript[99] of 1415 even though some of the detail is lost.

> To clean and heal wounds, it is good to pound this herb and to put honey through it ... pound this herb and put it in milk, and it will help with the spitting of blood and with the coughing that comes from hotness. If a plaster of this herb be put on a wound it will stop its bleeding. If the same herb be pounded and put through the

* Allen & Hatfield, *Medicinal Plants in Folk Tradition: An Ethnobotany of Britain & Ireland*, 248.

white of egg, it will help powerfully with a burn … if a linen cloth
be put in the juice of this, and it be put on the surface over the liver,
it will help with its swelling and pain. Ch. 52

Today, the young leaves may be used in salads, but they need to be
washed very well as they seem to harbour quite a lot of dust. When
they get bigger, they become too fibrous and may also cause a loose
bowel. Since they appear in the garden very early and are almost the
last to die back, it would be useful to ensure pride of place for this
plant in a herbaceous border, or vegetable patch, so that it is near at
hand in the event of a cut or burn. If one is not allergic to plantain, an
infusion of this herb may be used as skin lotion as it stimulates and
cleanses the skin.

Sweet violet/*Viola odorata*/*Sail cuach*

Spring brings that most inconspicuous and lovely flower, *viola odorata*,
and its heavenly scent is a real harbinger of the longer day. These flowers can be picked, made into syrup, or dried and candied. The advice
from tradition is to boil this herb and wash one's face and feet in the
water to obtain a good night's sleep. *Kitty Little's Book of Herbal Beauty*[194]
gives the following recipe for a foot bath of violet flowers. The water for
this foot bath would need to be comfortably hot.

> A violet foot bath containing ten or twelve flowers encourages
> sleep. Leave the flowers floating in the water. Wrap up warmly,
> then wriggle your bare toes in the foot bath for at least fifteen
> minutes. (p. 210)

Tradition also tells us that violets boiled in water stops drunkenness,
and if boiled in whey they are effective against pleurisy, pneumonia,
and other chest conditions. This herb is used more extensively in the
Ayurvedic medical system than in Europe, including Ireland.

Violet flowers can be used as garnish for cakes, pastries, poached
fruit and the syrup may soothe a cough. If growing violets, they like a
shady part of the garden and will spread if the area suits them. They can
in this instance be a good ground cover with the added advantage of
those lovely flowers in early spring.

It is possible then to integrate the different aspects of indigenous healing into one's life by adopting traditional rituals and outdoor activity, as well as connecting with our environment through use of plants and observation of the natural cycles of the earth.

Summer

Bealtaine/May 1st

Bealtaine, the first day of summer, is traditionally a particularly important day in the farming calendar, as the grass is growing well and all the animals can be turned out in the fields.

The bringing home of fresh flowers from the hedgerow is one of the many ways to celebrate the coming of summer and this task was usually done at dawn or just after it. A May bough may also be made and hung on the door. This could include holly, hazel, elder, or rowan, but in County Cork, the sycamore is the more usual choice. The whitethorn was never used, as it was considered unlucky to bring this into the house. In other parts of the country, a bush was set in front of a house on May Eve where it was decorated with eggshells and flowers. A bonfire was also lit, and the older people sat around chatting, while the younger generations sang and danced around the fire.

The dew of May morning was reputed to be beneficial to health and it was collected by placing a linen cloth on the ground. When this was soaked with the dew, the cloth was wrung out and the liquid collected and placed in a glass bottle. This was placed on a windowsill in the sun and left there for the summer. As the dregs fell to the bottom it was decanted into another bottle and this continued week on week until the water was completely clear, "The dew thus thoroughly purified looketh whitish, and keepeth good for a year or two after."[195] This liquid, as well as benefitting the skin, was also beneficial in the treatment of sore eyes and skin ailments.

The water taken from a well in May morning, *sgaith an tobair*, was potent for good or evil, and it was important to get the first water off the well that morning as it was this water that carried luck with it. Another tradition was walking around the farm, stopping at the four cardinal points, carrying the sacred herb, vervain, and some implements, to dig a sod and turn it to tilth. The land was then blessed with the *sgaith an tobair*. It was also the custom to light a candle and bless the hearth, the threshold, and the four corners of the house, as well as all its inhabitants, with the water taken from a well at Easter.

May was a critical time for sick people, and an illness contracted on May Eve was believed to be especially dangerous. This belief may have been due to May Eve being a time when the veil between this world and that of the fairy world was deemed to be very porous. Precautions, such as a piece of iron in one's pocket, were believed to offer protection against illnesses held to originate with the fairies, such as the evil eye and the fairy stroke. It was also discouraged to don summer clothes too early, and this was captured in the saying, "change not a clout 'til May is out."

May day was considered the best day for gathering herbs, and three meals of fresh young nettles, boiled until tender, were taken on consecutive days commencing on May day. Another way of taking nettle was to take three cups of the liquid in which they were boiled each day, commencing on May Day.[187]

So many rituals and activities are associated with *Bealtaine* that there is an embarrassment of riches in selecting a few for integrating the activities of our ancestors into our 21st century lives today.

- May is a time to take stock. The rigors of winter have passed, and summer sun and long days are now a reality. It is good to plan for the summer, to see where excess busyness can be shorn and where renewal of spirit can be obtained by relaxation, enjoying the countryside, and gardening.
- Decorate a shrub or tree in the garden or in the house with ribbons to celebrate the day.
- Have the first BBQ of the season.
- Pick some greenery and wildflowers for the house.
- Make a garland with fresh leaves of sycamore, elder, or rowan and hang on the door.
- Collect the dew from the grass as described above.
- If living near a source of fresh water, collect it on May morning
- Get a sprig of vervain and use it to bless the house and its inhabitants.
- Pick nettles and have them for dinner.
- Find out when the dog star appears in the sky again as this is when vervain should be harvested for the year ahead.
- Make a trip to the sea, countryside, or mountains on May Day.

St John's eve, June 23rd

Bonfires are associated with celebrations of the summer solstice and they are lit at sunset, which is after 10 pm. The first rays of dawn slip over the horizon as early 4 am on June 24th so it is one of those nights where there is an undercurrent of light throughout the night sky. If the day has been warm and sunny, the scene is set for a magical night outdoors.

In times gone by, prayers may have been said for a good harvest, as by this time all the farmer can do is wait. There is a custom associated with the community fire that could well be introduced again. A man, who has built a new house, will take red hot embers from the community fire to light the first fire in the new house. The new home was thus blessed by the *Teine Féil Eóin*/Fire of St John. If there is not a communal fire than a family BBQ and fire pit could be a twenty first century adaptation.

Herbs that were normally picked at this time, and before the end of June, were St. John's worth/*Hypericum perforatum*, Mugworth/*Artemesia vulgaris* and Yarrow/*Achillea millefolium*. Yarrow was deemed to ward off evil and for this reason was burned in the *Teine Féil Eóin*/Fire of St John.

Valuable food and plants in summer

Summer is the busiest time of the year in the garden and there is no time to spare if the many useful and beneficial plants are to be harvested and processed for the year ahead.

Nettles

In the NFCS,[196] Mrs Sheehan, Kilcolman, Co. Limerick told the collector that,

> Nettles were used for nourishing the blood, and for blood pressure in olden times. In order to prepare nettles for nourishing the blood, a person would have to boil the nettles in water for about a half an hour. The nettles would then be strained and eaten like cabbage.

The many benefits of nettles for health was also noted in Co. Kilkenny where the informant tells us that,[197]

NETTLES are good for people to eat during the month of May. "If we eat 'three feeds of nettles' during this month we will escape sickness during the year" is an old saying. Boiled like cabbage they should be. They purify the blood.

Elderflower/*Sambucus Nigra/Trom*

This is one of the most well-known and useful plants to be found in the hedgerows of the Irish countryside in late May and early June. Traditionally, a tea was made of the fresh flowers and Ita McDonagh from Co Galway tells us, "The elderflower and peppermint, taken in hot infusions frequently, is a great remedy for colds and influenza."[198]

Elderflower cordial is a refreshing drink that is easily made. The flowers for this cordial are best collected when some of the flowers are open but others are still in bud.

This is the my recipe but there are many variations.

Ingredients:

30 elderflowers
1.5 kg castor sugar
2 lemons
50 g citric acid
1 Campden tablets

Method:

- Bring the sugar and 2 litres of water to boil in a large saucepan. Stir until sugar is dissolved and leave to cool.
- Slice the lemons thinly and place in a large and very, clean bucket.
- Add the elderflower heads to the same bucket with the citric acid and Campden tablet.
- Pour the sugar syrup into the bucket and cover it loosely with a clean cloth.
- Leave 48 hours and then strain through muslin or a sieve.
- Bottle and store in the fridge.
- Dilute at a ratio of 1 part cordial to 5 parts still/sparkling water.

Elderflowers can also be frozen, and this is done by placing 20–30 flower heads in a bag. When needed, do not defrost but add directly to boiling water if making an infusion, or to the hot sugar syrup if making a cordial.

By freezing them they are to hand in the event of a cold or flu, where they can be added to a tea to help induce sweating, which is useful in the management of respiratory infections.

Selfheal/*Prunella vulgaris*/Lus an Chroidhe/Ceannabháin Beag

This herb is not mentioned frequently in the national folklore archives, but the accounts therein recommend its use for worms. It was also known as the herb of the heart (*Lus an Chroidhe*) and this use has now been supported by research where *Prunella* has been shown to reduce atherosclerosis or hardening of the arteries (in mice, at least). It was used more for staunching bleeding in England, but its more common use here was for fevers, especially in children.[199]

> This herb is used as a cure for a children's disease (adults take the disease too, but not as commonly as children). This disease is something in intensity like a fever and lasts twenty-one days. The malady is called the "Mionnéarach."

It was also used to heal tubercular coughs in counties Kildare, Laois, Carlow, and Offaly.[23] There is another use for this wonderful little plant and that is for *herpes simplex*. To resolve this viral infection, simply crush a leaf or the flower to the lesion and notice the immediate relief. To preserve for winter, make a strong infusion of the herb, reduce to a quarter and freeze in ice cube trays. Defrost a cube and bathe the area when required.

Mullein/Verbascum spp./Coinneal Mhuire/Lus Mór

Mullein was well known in Ireland and used extensively for tuberculosis. The following account by Ita Harlin shows a familiarity with its preparation and use.[200]

> Mullein is valued for coughs, and all affections of the lungs. For this purpose, make an infusion of one ounce of the dried leaves, boiled for ten minutes in a pint of milk. Strain carefully; for the minute hairs that cover the leaves are a most powerful irritant to the mouth and throat. Administer in small quantities three times a day. It has a pleasant taste.

Dried leaves smoked in cigarette form are said to relieve some forms of asthma.

For colic and catarrh an infusion of the flowers in water is beneficial.

Mullein flowers in olive oil exposed daily in a corked bottle to the sun are used in parts of the Continent for chilblains, earache, etc.

The leaves have also been used as a poultice for "running sores",[178] and an infusion of the leaves have been used in County Kerry to bathe areas affected by pain.[201]

> If any person has pains and could not be cured by any doctor and if he looked in the fields for a plant which is called Mullein plant and boiled it and rubbed the water to his body, it would cure him.

Even though there are many other plants awaiting attention in the summer, nettles, elderflower, selfheal, and mullein are particularly useful all the year round.

Autumn

Lughnasa

Lá Lughnasa takes place on August 1st and celebrates Lugh, a god of the Tuatha de Danann. Lugh rescued his people from oppression and won the secret of successful agriculture from the despot, Bres. The customs and traditions associated with *Imbolc, Bealtaine,* and *Samhain* are tied to the eve and day of their respective feasts, but the festivities of *Lughnasa* can vary from the last Sunday in July to after the first Sunday in August. In some instances, the *Lughnasa* festivities take place anytime in the two weeks either side of August 1st. *Lughnasa* also differs from the other quarter festivals in that it is a general gathering of people, not just a single household, and takes place outdoors, not within, or near, the home. The usual venues for these community gatherings were natural features such as heights, springs, lakes, or rivers.

Even though the traditions associated with *Lughnasa* may take place within a broader time frame, the *Lughnasa* festival is recognised as the commencement of Autumn with its shortening days and longer nights. It also heralds the work of harvesting the earth's bounty, so that there is sufficient stored to see households through the long winter. In days of yore, when meeting others was not as frequent as today, *Lughnasa* was a time for joy and revelry. The anxiety of watching over crops during the summer was over, and the first fruits of the year's work was evident in the new potato crop, and corn sheaves.

Reek Sunday

Mountain pilgrimages were, and are, an important feature of the celebrations of *Lughnasa* and the most well-known of these is Reek Sunday, which is the last Sunday in July, an occasion when as many as 20,000 people will climb Croagh Patrick, in County Mayo. This mountain is 2,500 feet high, and many pilgrims climb the rocky terrain of the reek in their bare feet. Even though it was originally a pre-Christian site, the mountain has long been associated with St Patrick, with the earliest written record of this pilgrimage dating from the 7th century. It was during his forty day fast on this mountain, then known as *Cruachán Aigle*, that Patrick fought with the demon-birds that encircled the mountain and blackened the sky. Ringing the bell that St Brigid had given him was to no avail but when he threw it at the birds, they vanished.[202] An ancient relic known as the *Clog Dubh,* or the black bell of St Patrick, was reputed to be the same bell that Patrick used to banish the birds, and until the latter half of the 19th century was brought to the Reek during the pilgrimage. The last keeper of the bell sold it to Sir William Wilde, father of Oscar, who presented it to the Royal Irish Academy, in Dublin. It may now be seen in the National Museum, Dublin.

In her mighty tome, *The Festival at Lughnasa,* Máire MacNéill counts seventy-eight hills where there were gatherings on the last Sunday of July or the first Sunday of August.[202] These occasions took the whole day and people gathered from a wide area to celebrate the harvest. Danaher[187] tells us that,

> On the last Sunday in July the people of Mountrath, Trumera, and the surrounding districts go up on the Slieve Bloom mountains, on to the slopes of Ard Erin. They bring with them food and spend the day on the mountain. (p. 170)

"Hurt" or whortle berry (*Vaccinium spp.)* picking was another favourite outing at this time and many a family brought home a bountiful harvest from the hills.

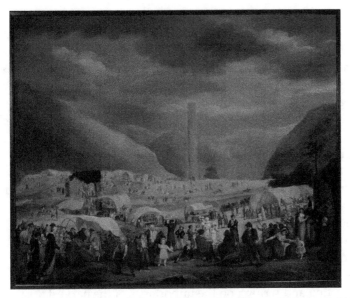

Pattern day at Glendalough from National Folklore Collection UCD.

Another favourite place to gather were lakes and rivers and, again, these were occasions for dancing, eating, and drinking as well as general merriment. It was also a favourite time for patterns (derived from the Irish, *patrun* or English, patron) at various wells associated with Saints and for fairs.

Puck fair

The most famous fair is probably Puck fair, held each year in Killorglin, Co. Kerry, on August 10th, 11th and 12th. It is a fair that can trace its roots back to 1603, and is a gathering associated with the Celtic festival of *Lughnasa*. The festival commences with the capture of a wild goat, Puck, who is then crowned king of the fair by a young girl, "Queen Puck." The girl is chosen from the final year in primary school, making her typically eleven to twelve years old. Once the coronation is complete, the trading and festivities commence with the first day being known as the Gathering Day, the second as the Fair Day and the third as the Scattering Day. At the end of the fair the goat is returned to the wild.

The months of August, September, and October are occupied with harvesting and storing food for the long winter ahead. It is more difficult today to be aware of the need for the harvest bounty to last for twelve months, but this is the harsh reality for many people worldwide as well as our forebears in Ireland. *Lughnasa* can be incorporated into our vision of a healthy lifestyle by incorporating the spiritual, physical, intellectual, and emotional aspects of the feast. Some of these activities may include,

- Climbing Croagh Patrick, or any suitable nearby mountain
- Visiting the National Museum to see St. Patrick's bell
- Locating and climbing some of the other pilgrimage sites, such as Mount Brandon, Co. Kerry, Slieve Donard in Co. Down, and Church Mountain, Co. Wicklow
- Visiting Puck fair
- Attending a local parish fair/show
- Taking a picnic to spend a day at a lake or river side
- Reflecting and writing on the importance of the harvest
- Deciding what foods are the most necessary to survive twelve months until the next harvest
- Harvesting and processing wild fruit for the winter, especially black-berries, wild strawberries, and damsons
- Listening to the sounds of the birds
- Noticing when the swallows leave and how they gather beforehand

Valuable food and plants in autumn

Autumn continues the "busyness" of summer, and there are many useful and beneficial plants to be harvested and processed for winter. The most important of these for the domestic medicine cabinet are:

- Yarrow
- Elderberry
- Marigold
- Marshmallow

Yarrow/Achillea millefolium/Lus na fola, Lus na gCluas, Athair Talmhan

Yarrow is one of the most useful herbs to have in the home medicine cabinet, and when it is in flower the upper two-thirds of it is gathered.

There is no need to cultivate it if ground is scarce, as it can be widely wildcrafted and is found on waste ground. Maloney[178] tells us that it was powdered and used as snuff to relieve a congestive headache, but its main use in Irish indigenous medicine is for stopping bleeding as the first Irish name suggests, herb (*lus*) of the blood (*fola*). Crushing the leaves and applying them to a bleeding cut or wound will cause the flow to stop within a very short space of time. A toothache may be relieved by either chewing the leaves or placing the chopped leaves in a pipe and smoking it. In 1938, Statia Kehoe tells us that, "yarrow … was known as the "herb of seven needs"[203] on account of its great healing power, and yarrow leaves are often sewn up in clothing as a protection against disease." James Gilchrist says,[204] "There is no better cure for a cold than yarrow and new milk. The yarrow is cut and boiled in the milk for half an hour. Then it is strained, and the milk is taken hot going to bed." A detailed account of how to prepare and use yarrow to alleviate rheumatism is given by Mrs Sheehan,[205]

> If a person suffers from Rheumatism, he gets a bunch of yarrow and boils the roots and stems of it. The yarrow is allowed to simmer over the fire for two days. It is then taken up and left aside. When required it is strained and half a cup is taken twice a day. A fresh supply is boiled after two or three days.

Current scientific research supports the use of yarrow as an antimicrobial and there are some preliminary studies to indicate that it may be a useful adjunct therapy in pancreatic cancer.[206] However, in the home, it needs to be dried and stored for the winter, and though drying it may not be a problem, storage may be. The best way to store dried herbs is to place them in brown paper bags in a press that will not succumb to any damp. An airing cupboard is ideal. A cardboard box packed with neatly labelled bags of herbs will not take up a lot of space in an airing cupboard and there is no danger of damp or mould getting near them. When needed, remove what you want and replace the rest until another time.

When to use yarrow

As already mentioned, yarrow is good for colds and this is because it reduces fever and induces sweating. It may be taken, as described in the NFSC, as a tea. Use 1 oz of the dried herb to one pint of water. Place the

herb in a ceramic tea pot and pour the boiling water over it. Infuse for
ten minutes and let it cool. Strain and drink the liquid freely at the onset
of a cold. The effectiveness of this tea is enhanced by the addition of
mint and elderflower. As a tea, yarrow may also be taken for digestive
upsets.

A yarrow salve is a useful remedy for cuts and scrapes. This is made
by drying a bunch of yarrow and when it is totally dry grinding it
coarsely. Place in a glass jar and cover with olive oil. Make sure that
the herb is well coated with the oil and leave in a sunny spot for two to
three weeks. After that, strain out the herb and add it to the compost.
Place the strained oil in a double boiler and heat gently. Add beeswax,
stirring all the time. The ratio of oil to wax is four to one. When the
wax is well incorporated, remove from heat and pour into small con-
tainers. Cover, label, and store in a cool dark place. It will keep for six
months and can be used for bleeding from wounds, minor cuts, burns,
and bites.

Yarrow should not be taken by pregnant or nursing mothers.

Elderberry/*Sambucus nigra*/*Caor throim*/*Ceireachán*

I have already spoken of the value of elder flower, and the berry is just
as useful. They should not be eaten raw as they can upset one's stomach. However, once cooked, they are both beneficial and delicious. They
may be added to tarts and made into jams and syrups.

Traditionally, the medicinal effects of elder have been known in
Europe since the time of Hippocrates and the leaves, flowers, and fruit
were all considered to have therapeutic value, with the leaves being used
to cool and soften swellings and wounds, and the bark to treat kidney
and urinary problems. Interestingly, black elder bark was considered
the "treatment of choice for grand mal or petit mal epilepsy."[207]

Today, Sidor and Gramza-Michalowsk, in their review of elderberry,
have this to say, "Elderberry … can greatly affect the course of disease
processes by counteracting oxidative stress, exerting beneficial effects
on blood pressure, glycaemia reduction, immune system stimulation,
anti-tumour potential … ."[208] It is, then, a fruit well worth harvesting
in the autumn. It also has the advantage that it can be grown in a small
area and coppiced regularly. It has proven to be effective in reducing
the severity of influenza A and B strains in patients and is the subject of
much research as both a functional food and a therapeutic agent.

Its effectiveness against respiratory infection is also evident in the NFSC where accounts of its use as food, wine, and medicine are recorded. A student in Clochar Lughbhaidh, Bundoran, Co. Donegal tells us that to make elderberry jelly, one must use, "one part, apples to three parts elderberry and lemons"[209] and Bernadette O'Hara tells us how the wine from this fruit was made.[210]

> Elderberry wine: first pluck the berries. when they are black. then put them in a bottle or jar along with some sugar and water and then cork them tight. then brew them under the ground for 10 days. when they are brewed take them up and strain the wine out of them. This wine is intoxicating.

As well as an enjoyable drink, this wine was also used for colds and drunk before going to bed.

A rather unusual use for elderberry is recounted by Peadar Mac Giolla Choinnigh who, tells us that the juice was mixed with soot to make ink for students in the hedge schools[211] and John Guihen, on the thirty first of March 1938, tells of another use for the plant:[212]

> Mrs Evans, Tarmon, Co. Leitrim has the cure of the burn. She first gets the inner bark of the elderberry Tree and boils it in unsalted butter along with some herbs, for about one hour. She then strains it through cheese cloth and puts it into little boxes. In a day or so it is like regular salve or ointment and can then be applied to any burn. After the burn is dressed, with the salve a few times, it is completely cured.

Another description of this cure, from July 19th, 1938, is as follows.[212]

> Elderberry makes a good ointment to heal a burn. The bark has to be scraped off and the green substance underneath has to be boiled along with cabbage and butter. It is then strained and when it cools it is quite firm.

The boiled bark of the elderberry is also used as poultice, "for all kinds of sores. The bark of the elderberry was also used in making ointment for cuts on horses' legs" and was deemed highly effective.[213]

The best way to harvest elderberries is as follows

- Pick the entire umbel of berries making sure there are not too many green fruits present.
- Strip the berries from the umbel using a fork.
- Weigh the quantity picked and freeze in small quantities if not able to process as tea, wine, jelly, or salve immediately.
- Make sure date and quantity are on the label.
- When needed, there is no need to defrost; simply process as required but do not eat uncooked.

Marigold/*Calendula officinalis*/Ór Mhuire

Marigold was used to give butter a deep yellow colour and used externally in the treatment of wounds, sprains, and bruises. Maloney[178] tells us that, internally, it was recommended as a uterine tonic. Ó Cuinn (1415) says that it has the ability to nourish against every poison, but it is better used fresh. This is not going to be possible during the winter, but it can be harvested every three to four days from May to late September, early October depending on the weather. Ó Cuinn[46] also suggests that using marigold in wine or ale is therapeutic to the liver and spleen, and when used as a tea for nine days it will relieve jaundice.

Within the NFCS there are accounts of marigold being used as a flavouring for soups, and as a sign of rain if the petals close during the day. Elizabeth White tells us that, "Marigold and hazel bark mixed is a cure for bruises, sprains, and cuts"[214] whereas, Mary Woods informs us that, "Chicken pox and measles were cured by drinking the juice of marigold flowers."[215] This must have been a popular cure for measles in Co. Kilkenny, as Alice Walsh, from Thomastown, was told by her father that, "Measles were cured by drinking the juice of a marigold."[216] In the same county, Danny Mc. Loughlin, from Mullinavat, gives more specific detail of how marigold was prepared;[217] "A remedy for measles [is] one ounce in a pint of boiling water. A tablespoon to be taken until the measles are well on the body." A similar recipe was recorded much further north, in Co. Longford, where an account from Killasona says that,[218] "MARIGOLD is a cure for measles and the infusion of one ounce in one pint of boiling water and one tablespoonful taken often until measles disappear."

A marigold infusion was also used in the treatment of fevers with accounts originating from different areas of the country. In Co.

Waterford, there is a record stating that, "The root of the marigold flowers are boiled for a couple of hours, and drunk for to cure fever because it promotes the perspiration, and the fever,"[219] and from Co. Sligo, we see its role again as a diaphoretic as, "The Marigold Flower is used for internal fevers and promotes perspiration."[220] The use of marigold in treating measles and fever has also been reported in a review paper from India on the importance of marigold as a medicinal crop for commercial cultivation[221] and a research paper from Iran notes that, "In France they commonly use it brewed to lower body temperature and perspiration as an effective tranquilizer."[222]

The most common use of marigold, in the home today, is as an anti-inflammatory and it may be used in two ways, an ointment or a compress.

A compress may be made by soaking a piece of cloth or swab in cold marigold tea. This can then be used for,

- Healing wounds, cuts, scrapes, scratches, and bites
- As an inflammatory in bruises and sprains
- Soothing sunburn

Made into an ointment it can be

- Applied to swollen varicose veins at least twice daily for three to four weeks.
- Used for nappy rash where it is a very effective remedy as it is both soothing and healing.

Marshmallow/ Althea officinalis/Leamhach

Marshmallow is the fourth herb that is important for the home medicine cabinet in the winter. There are over a hundred accounts of its use in the NFCS, and these include its use as a remedy for bronchitis and whooping cough, but it appears to have been more commonly used for healing sprains, cuts, and bruises.

Tessie Kielty from Irishtown, Co. Wexford tells us to,[223]

> Chop the leaf finely and put it in a pan of boiling fat (fresh lard).
> Put in a small piece of pure bee's wax.
> Strain the mixture and allow to cool.

This makes a very good ointment for cuts, sores, bruises etc.

Matt McGuiness from Raheny, Co. Dublin says, "that a cure for a sprain is, boil marshmallow and bathe the sprain with the water of the marsh-mallow"[224] and in an account from Co. Limerick it was the root that was used for the same purpose.

> If a person sprained his foot or his hand long ago, the old people
> got marshmallows and scraped the roots and applied them as a
> poultice to the sprains. When the marshmallows would fall off the
> sprains would be cured.[225]

The cures used for bronchitis originate from all over the country and we are told that, "when the leaves are brewed (like tea) it is known to cure the most obstinate cough."[226] is more detail given in volume 0764: 436 from Co. Longford, where both root and leaves are used.

> MARSHMALLOW leaves are an old-fashioned remedy for coughs,
> colds and whooping cough. An ounce of the leaves in one and a
> half pints of boiling water boiled down to one pint, makes a useful
> fomentation for inflamed wounds, boils, or abscesses.
>   ROOTS-four ounces of dried marshmallow roots put into five
> pints of water and boiled down to three pints, then strain, is consid-
> ered useful for bladder and kidney trouble.[227]

The reference to bladder and kidney trouble echoes the account in Ó Cuinn (1415) when he tells us that a "porridge made from this herb greatly reduces the pain of the urinary stone if drunken."

The confidence of people in plants, and the ability to accept and recognise that knowledge comes in many forms, is seen in the follow-ing account from Co. Roscommon.[228]

> Long ago a woman lay in bed with cancer. She was in terrible pain.
> The doctors could not relieve her. One night she had a vision and
> she saw bushes of marshmallow growing in a garden and a voice
> seemed to say, "If you desire relief from the pain, apply some leaves
> of the herb to the cancer."
>   When she wakened in the morning she spoke of the vision to her
> husband, and he immediately sent for the leaves. The leaves took
> away the pain and she lived a long time afterwards.

This account may have a factual basis, as modern research into the root of marshmallow has shown that it affects cell proliferation and may have potential as an anti-cancer remedy.[229]

Harvesting marshmallow

One of the problems with marshmallow leaves is that they are difficult to dry. Once dried, they also have a tendency to go mouldy unless great care is taken with their storage. One way of drying them is to pick them on a windy day and fill a net or muslin bag loosely with the leaves. Hang on a clothesline for two days if possible. Do not leave out overnight as they will absorb the moisture. This method gets the excess moisture out of the herb and it is then easier to dry them on a windowsill or in a green house. They have a tendency to get scorched very easily so care has to be taken. Once dried, crumble the leaves and store. Marshmallow is the one herb that almost justifies the purchase of a dehydrator and, if this herb becomes a staple of your home medicine cabinet, this purchase may be worthy of consideration.

The root is not usually a problem as it can be dug as needed in the winter. However, the root may not be as therapeutically effective in the spring as its energy will be moving up into the new growth. Other methods of preserving the root would be to freeze it after cleaning and cutting it up or making a glycerite, or syrup from it.

Having looked at the different events and plants that may be used during Autumn to connect us to our indigenous traditions, it is now time to explore the festivals and plants of winter.

Winter

Halloween

The first of November is the start of Winter and the festival of *Samhain* commences the evening before. November 1st is also the feast of All Hallows or All Saints and it is from this term that we derive the modern festivities associated with Hallwe'en or the eve of all Hallows.

In some areas this night was known as *púca* night or *oiche na sprideanna*, because of the widespread belief that the "good people" and the ghosts of the dead are abroad during the darkness. This festival is also looked upon as the end of the growing season as the *púca* spit on the blackberries and other wild fruit, so no fruit is deemed edible after this night. This belief marks a clear end to all harvesting and heralds the quietness of winter. Food offerings are left at the door for the fairies to ensure their favour for the coming year.[187]

It is on this night too that the souls of the unquiet dead return, and those who have wronged someone who has died, fear this night in case the injured party returns.

Hallowe'en is also a night of fun and games. The main work of the year is over and if the harvest has been good, there are sufficient stores for the year ahead. Traditionally, the eve of All Saints has been a day when no meat was eaten, so a favourite food was colcannon and there are many variations of this dish. It may be as simple as new potatoes mashed with new milk, seasoned with salt and served with butter, or the potatoes may be mixed with cooked cabbage and finely chopped raw onion, which is then seasoned with salt and pepper only. From Co. Galway we are told that,

> From the earliest times it has been the custom in this district to make colcannon for Halloween. The first plate of this is kept for the fairies lest they should [visit], while changing from their Summer residence to their Winter home. No salt should be put on their portion. Colcannon is made on this night also to commemorate the end of the digging of the potatoes.[230]

This was also a night when family members who had died might revisit their home. This account from Co. Cavan indicates that this was not a cause for fear but simply an acknowledgement that the dead may like to return to their former dwelling.

> The souls in Purgatory were supposed to be let loose on this night, so as to return to the homes of their living relatives. Many of the old people would not bolt the doors on this night. The hearth would be cleanly swept, a fire left burning, and a supper left ready for the dead.[231]

Danaher[187] gives an even more comprehensive account from County Tyrone of this belief, but it is for All Souls' Eve, November 1st.

> All Souls Eve is sacred to the memory of the departed. After the floor has been swept and a good fire put down on the hearth, the

family retires early, leaving the door unlatched and a bowl of spring water on the table, so that any relative who had died may find a place prepared for him at his own fireside. On that one night in the year the souls of the dead are loosed and have liberty to visit their former homes … In parts of County Limerick, a table was laid with a place for each of the dead, and the poker and tongs placed in the shape of a cross on the heartstone.

The eating of colcannon, the possible return of the departed, and the "Good people," feature in this account from Edengora, Co. Meath.

On HALLOW EVE NIGHT the 31st October apples and nuts and sweet cakes are eaten. On this night, the old people were afraid to leave their houses after dark as they believed that all the departed spirits were free to roam about and to come back to the houses they once inhabited. Colcannon, that is mashed potatoes and butter was eaten also on that night and when going to bed the woman of the house left some colcannon on a plate for the "Good people" as the spirits were called.[232]

Barm brack was also eaten on this night, and the finding of the pea, bean, rag, stick, and coin, was an occasion for merriment as well as the beginning of the many other festivities associated with this night. Some of these amusements are described by Patrick Coleman from Blarney, Co. Cork, as follows.

Hallowe'en night, or "snap—apple" night, is a great night in Ireland. At teatime that night the barm brack is cut and each member of the family takes a slice. There is great fun and excitement to see who will get the slice with the ring in it. It is said, whoever gets the ring is sure to get married within the next twelve months. The barm brack also contains the pea, bean, stick, and rag. When tea is over "snap—apple" starts. A tub half—full of water is placed in the middle of the kitchen, and the apples are put into it. Then each person comes along in turn and tries to snap an apple from the tub with his mouth. This causes great fun because the apple recedes from the person going after it, and usually results in the person getting half smothered in the water.[233]

We are told from Co. Waterford that, "The person who gets the ring is said to get married soon. He who gets the pea will have poverty. He who gets the rag is said to be in rags for a year. He who gets the stick is to beat his wife." The same informant tells of other divination ceremonies.

> Clay Water-Ring. The woman of the house gets three saucers and she puts a ring into one of them and she puts water into another, and she puts clay into the third saucer. Then she blindfolds a person and if he touches the saucer with the ring in it, he will be married before twelve months. If he touches the saucer with the water in it, he will cross water before twelve months. If he has the misfortune to touch the clay it is said that he will be buried before twelve months.[234]

These amusements are in addition to dressing up, and Henry Byrne, from Fairyhouse, Co. Meath tells us. "Many boys and girls dress themselves up on the Hallow Eve night. They go around from house to house singing and dancing and they get apples and nuts, and even money in some houses."[235]

Many of these traditions may be incorporated into life today, and by doing so we are acknowledging our forebears, the inevitability of death, and the possibility of an "other world." Rather, than leaving a meal overnight for those who have died it may be more positive to lay a place at table for those who have died recently. By doing this it provides an opportunity to talk about grief, to recall times of joy or sadness, and to honour their presence in our memories. It is also an opportunity to make colcannon and barm brack as well as practising divination.

November 2nd is All Souls Day and is sacred to the memory of the dead. Many people visit their family burial sites on this day. It was also customary to light a candle in the home for those who had died and often this candle was allowed burn itself out rather than be quenched. Leaving a candle to burn out is a vivid and palpable reminder that the natural end to life is death. This belief in the souls of the dead being loosed on this day crossed over into the belief that one's dead relations would come to your aid if you were in any danger on this day.

Valuable food and plants in winter

Between Halloween and the rush of Christmas there are some useful roots to dig in the garden. It is also an opportunity to see if there are any hazel nuts left on the trees, but these are usually picked in October with the last of the apple and pear crops. The traditional time for picking roots is during the waning two weeks after the November full moon. This is often the last waning moon before the December solstice and, even if there is another waning moon, it will be near to Christmas and in the middle of the preparations for this festival. It is even better if there has been a frost before harvesting roots as the cold causes the complex starches in the root to convert to sugar. This makes them much sweeter and easier to digest. Among the roots to harvest are:

Marshmallow/Althea officinalis/Leamhach

This herb has been discussed previously but now is the time to dig the roots. They need to be washed thoroughly and then sliced into strips. Lay them on a tray and place in a very cool oven until dry. Alternatively, place them above a radiator and the ascending air will help the drying process. In 1938, Eibhlín Ní Liathán from Co. Kilkenny tells us the, "dried roots boiled in milk will cure the whooping cough,"[236] whereas Nora Mc Nicholas just says, "The marshmallow is boiled, and the juice is drunk."[237]

Comfrey/Symphytum officinalis/Lus na gCnamh mBriste

In 1415, Ó Cuinn tells us that comfrey "has the ability to join and consolidate the bones" and accounts from Co. Leitrim in 1938 indicate that this use for comfrey was still well known because, "Comfrey roots will cure the leg of a horse or cow if broken. The roots are to be mashed up and put to the broken part."[238] From Co. Galway there is another account saying it was used for poultry: "Its roots when pounded up makes a sticking mass and used to be used by the old people with splints for setting broken legs of ducks, geese, etc."[239]

This account from Co. Clare gives the detail of how comfrey was prepared.

> "Comfrey" paste. Used for sprains. The "comfrey" plant has a large leaf like that of rhubarb and a long tapering root like that of a parsnip. The root is scraped, and the juicy exterior is made into paste which is put on a cloth and placed on the affected part. This "cure" is still largely practiced.[240]

From these accounts it is evident that comfrey was not made into a salve but dug up and prepared as needed, which suggests it needs its own permanent place in the garden. Even though comfrey should only be used externally, it is especially useful for both muscle and joint pain being both anti-inflammatory and pain relieving. It is no longer given internally, or put on broken skin, due to it containing pyrrolizidine alkaloids which are damaging to the liver.[241]

Burdock/Arctium lappa/Cnadán

Marshmallow deals with coughs and comfrey with bones, but the third root, burdock, has, many different uses recorded in the NFCS. Ó Cuinn (1415) has versatile uses for this herb also, including using it for stopping "the spitting of blood" and "if the roots of this herb be boiled in wine it will help with dysentery." Boiling it in wine also helps with urinary stones and if a salve is made of the root and herb using pig lard it will break and ripen boils. Myles Duffy from Virginia, Co. Cavan says that "Burdock cleans the blood and it is also used for kidney complaints."[242] The use for kidney complaints echoes the 15th century manuscript, but the 1938 record does not tell us how burdock was prepared. There are accounts from many parts of the country telling us that burdock was good for "purifying the blood,"[243] and on the 18th of May 1938, an informant tells us, "The 'Burdock' seed is noted as one of the best blood purifiers and is often used with other herbs for other purposes."[244] Its use for kidney trouble and skin disease is noted in Co. Louth, "The burdock spreads quickly and its roots have a cure for kidney trouble and skin disease."[245] It was also used for burns, "Burdock leaves are boiled and placed on a burn,"[246] and we are told from a student in Lowertown, Co. Cork how to prepare it to bring out measles, "BURDOCK was used to PUT OUT MEASLES. The root of it was first got, the skin was taken off of it then, and the root was boiled until all the juice left it, sugar candy used be boiled with the juice to put a sweet taste in it."[247]

Modern research has found ingredients in burdock that support its ability to improve skin quality and cure skin problems such as eczema, as well as compounds that have an inhibitory effect on tumours.[248] Its anti-inflammatory effects have also been noted, with more efficacy obtained in the root than the leaves. One of the problems associated with harvesting burdock in the wild is that it resembles the belladonna nightshade plants, and these are highly poisonous. Unfortunately, they often grow together so it is not recommended to wildcraft burdock. If needed, it is better to obtain it from a health food shop or pharmacy.

Dandelion root/*Taraxacum officinalis radix*/*Caisearbhán*

Even though dandelions are considered a weed by most people they have important medicinal features, and the NFCS documents four areas of use. These include an account from Mary Woods, Thomastown, Co. Kilkenny for biliousness, "Dandelion root steeped in water and strained was used as a medicine for biliousness"[249] and an account from Co. Limerick for lung trouble, "DANDELION root was dug, cleaned, and drawn like tea. It is a cure for lung trouble."[250] An account from Co. Mayo mentions its efficacy in both rheumatism and chest troubles, "The juice of a dandelion root boiled [and] taken every morning is a cure for rheumatism and is very good for chest diseases,"[251] and an account from Co. Wexford tells us how to prepare dandelion root for this purpose; "Dandelion root dried and cleaned and when stewed on water was used with success and in case of Rheumatism a wine glass full to be taken each morning."[252] There are accounts, also, of its effectiveness in kidney and liver trouble, "The dandelion root is used to cure kidney and liver complaints,"[253] but there are differences in how to prepare it. Mrs, Tarpey says to boil it in milk, "The cure for kidney trouble is the dandelion root boiled with milk added"[254] and an account from Co. Kilkenny tells us that, "Dandelion Root drawn like tea was used for liver and kidney trouble."[255] However, tea has milk added to it so that may also include the added milk mentioned by Mrs Tarpey.

Modern research has shown that all parts of the dandelion are highly nutritious, and it contains an impressive array of vitamins and minerals as well as fibre. The pharmacological properties of dandelion have shown it to be useful in many diseases, including its possible use in the management of Diabetes type two,[256] even though this use has not been recorded as a folk remedy anywhere in the UK, and only one instance in Ireland, in Co. Kilkenny.[23] Similarly, Allen and Hatfield noted no account of dandelion being used to treat cancer anywhere in these islands except for one account in Co. Carlow. Yet, the NFCS gives a quite detailed account from Breaghy, Co. Sligo.

> There are two types of cancer- running cancer and dry cancer. For running cancer there is no known cure but old people give the

following cure for dry cancer: - Some near relation of the person suffering from the disease must dig a few roots of dandelion and squeeze the juice out of them. Then this juice must be rubbed to the sore occasionally and after some time it will disappear.[257]

It is evident from this account that it is an external cancer and a plaster was the more typical cure used for these types of cancer. Whether dandelion was one of the herbs used in any of these plasters we don't know, as the formulae have always been kept secret. What is unusual, given the few references to the use of dandelion in vernacular medicine, is that modern scientific research sees dandelion as a promising novel anti-cancer agent in breast and prostate cancer[258] but then again, science is only discovering what Read has already suggested in "The Chirurgical Lectures of Tumors and Ulcers" written in 1635.[259]

Willow/*Salix alba*/*Sailleach*

November is also the time to harvest "sally rods" for weaving into baskets, making wattle fences, or even living garden sculptures and children's playhouses. John McCarthy from Anablaha, Co. Kerry says to pick the sally rods during the new moon.

> The work is done by hand by men during the long winter nights. The baskets are made from the twigs of a certain willow tree. The twigs are cut during a dark moon as the rods are supposed to be tougher then than when [?] at any other time.[260]

This account from Co. Monaghan tells us how to use a sally rod for getting rid of warts. "Get a piece of a willow-tree and put it in the fire. When it is lit, let the resin which will flow out at the other end to drop on to the wart."[261]

A more interesting cure comes from Mullingar, Co. Westmeath, where the sally rods are burnt until there is only ash left. This ash is mixed with white of egg and the resulting mixture is used to treat ringworm.[262, 263] This may be effective as the bark (of white willow) contains *salicin*, which was originally isolated from the tannins in willow in 1828, was further purified in 1829, manufactured on a large scale by the turn of the 20th century and is known to us today as Aspirin.

One of the easiest ways to experiment with willow crafts, such as basket making, is to stick ten strong willow rods in the ground about eight cm apart. Weave lighter rods through them until the desired height is reached and then pull up the entire structure. Turn it over and now weave between the rods that were stuck in the ground to give a base to the circle. So even though November may be a wet and windy month there is ample opportunity to practise forgotten skills in preparation for Christmas.

Christmas

It was a time of preparation for Christmas between the harvesting of roots in November and December 24th. This period also included the four weeks of Advent, and in former times this was a time of fasting in preparation for the great feast. In terms of health, fasting is beneficial as it fights inflammation, promotes blood sugar control by reducing insulin resistance, and of course helps to control obesity.[263] Periods of calorific restriction not only benefitted health, but also helped to regulate the consumption of the precious harvest during the long winter. The fasting during advent ends with a feast that celebrates the turn of the year, and the end of the short days and long nights.

Christmas today continues the core values of the feast, which is the gathering of family, friends, and community to celebrate the beginning of the new solar year. In the past, decorations consisted of holly, with berries if possible, and ivy. The big shopping for the meal was called "bringing home the Christmas" and a custom, which has mostly died out, was the shopkeeper giving a present to his customers in thanks for their custom during the year. Before the establishment of turkey as the centrepiece of the dinner table, roast beef held the honour.[187]

A very important custom on Christmas Eve is the lighting of the Christmas candle. This is a red candle, placed in a jar and lit by the youngest member of the family. This is then used to light other candles, all of which are placed in the windows to show Mary and Joseph, who found no place to stay in Bethlehem, that they would be welcome to stay. It was, and is, still customary to cut the Christmas cake, and serve tea and punch, after the lighting of the candles, thus signalling the commencement of the festivities.

Where Christmas Day was a day for family only, St Stephen's Day was a day for going out and about, or if staying at home to expect a visit from groups of "Wren boys." In times of yore this involved killing a wren, or finding a dead one, and placing it in a holly bush, which was then ceremoniously carried over the shoulder of the lead wren boy or Captain. The youngsters would visit each house in the countryside, singing the wren song.

> The wren, the wren the king of all birds,
> on Stephen's Day was caught in the furze
> Although he is little, his family is grate,
> Put your hand in your pocket and give us a trate.

The song is longer than this, but it generally faded away once the request for a treat was sung. Having a jar full of coins for the "Wran Boys" was one of many tasks that had to be remembered before retiring on Christmas Day, as the first group could arrive early on the day to ensure they gathered enough treats to celebrate the spending of it later. In Dingle today, the wren celebrations are highly organised, with different teams dressed in elaborate costumes of straw parading through the streets from early morning before retiring to the pubs afterwards. The main outdoor activities on this day include horse racing, walking, bowling, and shooting for gun club members, but it may also be a day of quiet recovery after the indulgence of Christmas Day. Even though we continue to celebrate Christmas today, it has become very commercial, and some useful, health-giving aspects that we may draw from tradition are,

- A period of fasting before Christmas
- A definite start and finish to Christmas shopping
- Using holly and ivy for decorations
- Lighting the Christmas candle
- Joining a wran group if there is one in your area or joining in the Dingle celebrations on social media
- Going to the races on Stephen's Day

January

New Year's Eve is a relatively new festival in Ireland as the Gregorian calendar was not adopted here until 1752, but divination of weather or other events on this day gave an indication of what the future year would hold. January 6th was, and is, known as *Nollaig na mBan* or Women's Christmas. The celebrations were not as lavish as Christmas Day, with lighter and more dainty food, such as cake and wine, being served. Today, many women will dine out with their friends or family and see it as a day of relaxation after the stress and strain of Christmas.

On January 7th the Christmas decorations were removed but Danaher[187] tells us that the withered greenery was saved to be burned to heat the pancake griddle on Shrove Tuesday. As February 1st commences the agricultural year, January is also a time for planning. It is the time to look forward, as the lengthening day is not yet noticeable, so there is an opportunity to plan the clearing, and planting for the year ahead. By following the four seasons in their natural rhythm it gives an opportunity to appreciate one's place in the natural order of life. It also allows us to integrate emotional, intellectual, spiritual, and physical health-giving opportunities into the annual round of the sun, thus continuing the *deiseal* tradition of our ancestors.

CHAPTER 5

Conclusion

E very day, people make health choices. These can range from a particular diet, to exercise, to medication. However, the means we take to ensure our health is governed by the society and culture in which we live. The options we have when faced with ill health will be determined, on the one hand, by what therapies are available in our society, and on the other, by our own understanding and knowledge of these same therapies. "Soul retrieval," as a therapy, will not be a treatment option in the event of severe psychological and physical trauma resulting in "soul flight," if one does not believe in, or consider, "soul flight" as a possible diagnosis in the first instance.

Whether one lives in a skyscraper in New York, or the depths of the Amazon, any illness requires diagnosis, prognosis, and treatment, and this may be carried out by a medicine man in a white coat with a stethoscope, or a medicine man in coloured robes with divination methods. Both medicine men are products of the medical system they have inherited, be it biomedicine or indigenous medicine. Biomedicine is the child of the scientific revolution initiated by Descartes and Bacon, among others, and further fastened by the subsequent success of scientific achievements. It is based on evidence that can be seen and measured and if this is not possible, the item under discussion does not exist as a problem,

129

or as a solution. This often rules out the effects of emotional or spiritual malaise on ill health unless the effects of this malaise can be measured and reproduced. Indigenous medicine, on the other hand, is governed by the belief that illness may be caused by many factors, including one's emotions, social situation, and even the spirit world.

Ireland's practitioners of vernacular medicine are generally known as the people "with a cure" and are, so to speak, hidden in plain sight throughout the country. Their cure is known to those they have helped, and knowledge of their healing ability is passed on by word-of-mouth. Very rarely does money change hands, but a donation is often proffered. There are different divisions within Irish vernacular medicine such as, physical manipulation, bonesetting, charms, prayers, and rituals; for example, the charm for stopping bleeding, and herbal cures for tuberculosis or shingles.

Tantalising glimpses of Ireland's indigenous medicine are portrayed in our myths and legends which may be gleaned from the *Lebor Gabhála Érenn*. There are accounts of psycho-somatic illnesses in the stories of Ailill and Covac, of herbal baths to heal the wounded at the battle of Moytura, and the use of cupping horns to heal the old unhealed wound on Cailte's leg. These descriptions give some indication of the range of therapies available. The advent of Christianity illustrates how health was perceived to be the result of a virtuous life, and ill health a punishment by the divine for wrongdoing. *The Annals* offer us a more objective insight into the causes of ill health during this time, as they record adverse weather being followed by famine disease and plague. The law texts, *Bretha Crólige* and *Bretha Dian Chécht* (Déin Chécht) tell us about the practice of medicine, the payments due to physicians, the compensation due to the affected party in the event of injury, the requirements for the hospital location, and the diet for patients. We are told that the three errors in nursing are leaving a patient without food, negligent medical care, and not organizing a substitute to do his work, while he is ill.

The extensive corpus of medical manuscripts between 1400 and 1700 point to the efforts of the Irish hereditary medical families to bring the new medical knowledge being taught in Europe to Irish medical schools. Because it was so different to the oral tradition hitherto taught, it necessitated the translation of the Latin texts into Irish, as well as the transcription of these texts. The hereditary medical families enjoyed considerable status and prestige, and being a physician attached to one of the great Irish families was well rewarded in terms of land and renu-meration. With the demise of the old Gaelic order, and the imposition of a new political establishment in the 17th century, this medical class went abroad, retrained, or adapted to the new political situation. Some of the current practitioners of vernacular medicine maintain their cure has been in the family for nine to ten generations, which may indicate the dissemination of the learned medical knowledge to the broader community in the political maelstrom of the 17th century. An examina-tion of the NFC and the NFCS also indicates the dissemination of plant knowledge among people via herbals available in Ireland from the 17th century, including those by Culpeper (1653), Threkeld (1726), and Keogh (1736). The NFC and the NFCS also point to the erosion of this knowledge, as valuable herbs are now, oftentimes, just called weeds.

This erosion of knowledge commenced in the 19th century, and there are many factors that may account for this. These possible fac-tors include the advent of primary school education in 1831, where the medium of teaching was English only, the Great Famine of the 1840s, increased emigration after the famine, the strengthened influence of the Roman Catholic Church, the decline in the speaking of Irish, and stem-ming from this, the loss of the "grandmother factor" because grandpar-ents could not communicate with their grandchildren through English. These many influences led, by the end of the 19th century and the early 20th century, to a social and cultural hegemony, where the Irish middle classes adopted the Victorian values and worldview prevailing then in Ireland. This change in worldview goes some way in explaining Ó Súilleabháin's description of Irish indigenous medicine in 1942, as a "large body of superstitious belief and practice ... this was especially so before the development of medicine as a science."[34] There were nascent attempts to establish scientific research and herb growing in the early 20th century, but these were based on developing an industry based on only one facet of Irish vernacular medicine, namely the plants.

Moore and McLean,[264] in their survey of two communities in Ireland, observed that traditional cures continued to be used if they were con-sidered to be effective, thus manifesting the functional choices people make every day regarding the therapeutic options open to them.

It is difficult for people who have no knowledge of the therapeu-tic choices within Irish indigenous medicine to adopt them, especially charms, prayers, and rituals, but it is possible to accept the four pillars that comprise health within this tradition. These are emotions, reason, spirituality, and physical exercise, all of which may be incorporated today into one's lifestyle. The most wholesome way of doing this is to live life according to the rhythms of the Irish calendar year, where the unfolding of the seasons, *Imbolc, Bealtaine, Lughnasa and Samhain*, may form the warp and weft of family celebrations, and country pursuits, thus integrating indigenous knowledge seamlessly into routine and daily life.

BIBLIOGRAPHY

1. Keating, Geoffrey, *The History of Ireland, 1634.* Translated and preface by David Comyn, Patrick S. Dinneen. Cork: UCC, Corpus of Electronic Texts Edition. (CELT) https://celt.ucc.ie//published/T100054/index. html: 2010.
2. Gray, Elizabeth, *Cath Maige Tuired: The Second Battle of Mag Tuired.* Kildare: Irish Texts Society 1982.
3. Sheehan, Áine, "Locating the Gaelic medical families in Elizabethan Ireland", in *Early Modern Ireland and the World of Medicine: Practitioners, Collectors and Contexts, edited by* J. Cunningham, 20–38, Manchester: Manchester University Press, 2019.
4. Ó Tuathaigh, Gearóid, *I mBéal an Bháis: The Great Famine and the Language Shift in Nineteenth-Century Ireland.* Cork. Cork University Press 2015
5. Larkin, Emmet, "Church, State, and Nation in Modern Ireland," *The American Historical Review,* vol. 80, no. 5 (Dec. 1975), pp. 1244–1276.
6. Konadu, Kwasi, *Indigenous Medicine and Knowledge in African Society.* New York: Routledge, 2007.
7. Blair O'Connor, Bonnie, *Healing Traditions: Alternative Medicine and the Health Professions.* Philadelphia: University of Pennsylvania, 1995.
8. WHO, *WHO Traditional Medicine Strategy 2014–2023.* 2014, WHO: http://www.who.int/medicines/publications/traditional/trm_ strategy14_23/en/.

9. Alver, Bente Gullveig, and Torunn Selberg, "Folk Medicine as Part of a Larger Concept Complex," in *New Perspectives on Witchcraft, Magic and Demonology,* edited by B.P. Levack. 1–25, New York: Routledge, 2001.

10. Iaccarino, Maurizio. "Science and Culture." *EMBO Reports* (European Molecular Biology Organisation), vol. 4, Issue 3, (March, 2003): 220–223. Available at https://doi.org/10.1038/sj.embor.embor781

11. Mazzocchi, Fulvio. "Western Science and Traditional Knowledge." *EMBO Reports* (European Molecular Biology Organisation), vol. 7, Issue 5, (May 2006): 463–466. Available at, https://www.ncbi.nlm.nih.gov/pmc/articles/PMC1479546/

12. Bodeker, Gerard and Kishan Kariippanon. "Traditional Medicine and Indigenous Health in Indigenous Hands." in *Oxford Research Encyclopedia of Global Public Health.* Oxford: Oxford University Press, 2020.

13. WIPO. *Panel of Indigenous and Local Communities—Lost in Transition: Traditional Healers of South East Nigeria and the Delegitimization of Traditional Knowledge and Cultural Expressions in the Age of Modernity.* Document Prepared by Mr. Ikechi MGBEOJI, Associate Professor, Osgood Hall Law School, Toronto. WIPO/GRTKF/IC/10/INF/5(D). Geneva: World Intellectual Property Organisation, 2006.

14. Kimball, Roger. "What's left of Descartes." *The New Criterion,* vol. 13, no. 10 (June 1995).

15. Ó Giolláin, Diarmuid. *Locating Irish Folklore: Tradition, Modernity, Identity.* Cork: Cork University Press, 2000.

16. Valussi, Marco. *A Translation and Discussion of One Recipe in a 14th century Italian antidotarium.* Online: Academia Edu. no date. https://www.academia.edu/2302809/A_translation_and_discussion_of_one_recipe_in_a_14th_century_italian_antidotarium

17. Capra, Fritjof. *The Turning Point: Science, Society and the Rising Culture.,* New York: Simon & Schuster, 1982.

18. Famousscientists.org *"René Descartes."* https://www.famousscientists.org/rene-descartes/ Accessed 20th May 2020.

19. Descartes, René. Discourse on Method. *Vol. XXXIV, Part 1. The Harvard Classics.* Edited by P.F. Collier & Son, 1909–14; New York: Bartleby.com, 2001. www.bartleby.com/34/1/

20. Waldstein, Anna, and Cameron Adams. "The Interface between Medical Anthropology and Medical Ethnobiology." *The Journal of the Royal Anthropological Institute,* vol. 12 (2006): 95–118.

21. Fantoni, Francesco., et al., "Current concepts on the functional somatic syndromes and temporomandibular disorders." *Stomatologija,* Baltic Dental and Maxillofacial Journal, vol. 9, issue 1, (2007): 3–9.

22. Lu, Mingjun. "Cosmo-Metaphysics: The Origin of the Universe in Aristotelian and Chinese Philosophy," *Dao,* vol. 16, (November 2017): 465–482.

23. Allen, David and Gabrielle Hatfield, *Medicinal Plants in Folk Tradition: An Ethnobotany of Britain & Ireland*. Cambridge: Timber Press, 2004.

24. Yoder, Don. "Folk Medicine." in *Folklore and Folklife: an Introduction*, Edited by R.M. Dorsan, 191–216, Chicago: University of Chicago Press, 1972.

25. Park, Katherine. *Doctors and Medicine in Early Renaissance Florence.* Princeton, New Jersey: Princeton University Press, 1985.

26. Battiste, Marie. *Reclaiming Indigenous Voice and Vision*. Vancouver: University of British Colombia Press, 2000.

27. Ruddle, Kenneth and Ray Chesterfield, *Education for Traditional Food Procurement in the Orinoco Delta*. Berkley: University of California Press, 1977.

28. McGregor, Deborah. "Traditional Ecological Knowledge." *Ideas: the Arts and Science Review*, vol. 3, no. 1, (Spring 2006): Faculty of Arts & Science, University of Toronto.

29. Wilde, Lady. *Ancient Legends, Mystic Charms, and Superstitions of Ireland.* London: Ward & Downey. 1888 (1971 ed.).

30. Coxhead, Elizabeth. "Foreward." in *Visions & Beliefs in the West of Ireland*, 5–8 Gerrards Cross, Buckinghamshire: Colin Smyth 1979 edition, (1920).

31. Wood-Martin, William Gregory. *Traces of the Elder Faiths in Ireland: A Folklore Sketch: A Handbook of Irish Pre-Christian Traditions.* Miami: Hard Press, 2013, (1902, London: Longmans Green and Co.)

32. Uí Ógáin, Ríonach and Tom Sherlock, eds. *The Otherworld. Music & Song from Irish Tradition.* Baile Átha Cliath: Four Courts Press, 2012.

33. Gregory, Augusta. *Visions & Beliefs in the West of Ireland.* Gerrards Cross, Buckinghamshire: Colin Smyth Ltd. 1979 edition (1920).

34. Ó Súilleabháin, Sean. *A Handbook of Irish Folklore*, London: Herbert Jenkins, 1963.

35. Evans, Estyn. *Irish Folk Ways*, London: Routledge & Kegan Paul, 1957 (1967 edition).

36. Bascom, William. "The Forms of Folklore: Prose Narratives." *The Journal of American Folklore*, vol. 78, no. 307 (Jan–March 1965): 3–20.

37. Agarwal, A. and R. Agarwal. "The practice and Tradition of Bonesetting." *Education for Health*, vol. 23 issue 1 (2010): 1–8.

38. Grenier, Louise, *Working with Indigenous Knowledge a Guide for Researchers*: Ottawa: International Development Research Centre (IDRC), 1998.

39. Hill, Dawn Martin. *Traditional Medicine in Contemporary Contexts: Protecting and Respecting Indigenous Knowledge and Medicine.* Ottawa, ON: National Aboriginal Health Organisaton, 2003. Available at www.naho.ca/documents/naho/english/pdf/research_tradition.pd...

40. Binchy, Daniel A., "Bretha Crólige" *Ériu*, vol. 12, (1938): 1–77.

41. Binchy, Daniel A., "The Leech in Ancient Ireland," in *What's Past is Prologue. A Retrospect of Irish Medicine*, edited by W. Doolin and O. Fitzgerald, 5–9. Dublin:, Monument Press, 1952.
42. Kelly, Ferfgus. "Medicine and Early Irish Law." *Irish Journal of Medical Science*, vol. 170 (2001) 71–76.
43. Nic Dhonnchadha, Aoibheann. "Medical Writing in Irish." *Irish Journal of Medical Science*, vol. 169, no. 3 (2000): 217–220.
44. Ó Crualaoich, Gearóid, *The Book of the Cailleach*. Cork: Cork University Press, 2003.
45. Iyioha, Irehobhude O, and Remigius N. Nwabueze, eds. *Comparative Health Law and Policy. Critical Perspectives on Nigerian and Global Health Law*. London: Ashgate, 2015.
46. Lock, Margaret and Vinh-Kim Nguyen, *An Anthropology of Biomedicne*. Oxford: Wiley-Blackwell, 2010.
47. Kleinman, Arthur and Peter Benson "Anthropology in the Clinic: The Problem of Cultural Competency and How to Fix It." *PLoS Medicine*, vol. 3 no. 10 (2006): 1673–1676. Available at https://journals.plos.org/plosmedicine/article?id=10.1371/journal.pmed.0030294
48. Battiste, Marie and James Youngblood (Sa'ke'j) Henderson., *Protecting Indigenous Knowledge and Heritage: A Global Challenge*. Saskatoon: Purich Press, 2000.
49. Kleinman, Arthur. *The Illness Narratives. Suffering, Healing, and the Human Condition*. New York: Basic Books, 1988.
50. Kleinman, Arthur. *Patients and Healers in the Context of Culture*. Berkeley: California University Press, 1980.
51. Kleinman, Arthur. "Medicine's symbolic reality." *Inquiry*, vol. 16, issue 1–4 (1973): 206–213.
52. Nolan, Peter W., "Folk Medicine in Rural Ireland." *Folk Life*, vol. 27, issue 1 (1988): 44–56.
53. Logan, Patrick. *Irish Country Cures*. Belfast: Appletree Press, 1981.
54. Hull, Eleanor, "The Ancient Hymn-Charms of Ireland." *Folklore*, vol. 21, no. 4 (1910): 417–446.
55. Mauss, Marcel. *The Gift*. London: Routledge. 1954, (2002 classic edition).
56. Ray, Celeste, "The Sacred and the Body Politic at Ireland's Holy Wells." *International Social Science Journal*, vol. 62, no. 205–206 (2011): 271–285.
57. Nugent, Louise. *Stories of Faith. Stories of Pilgrimage from Medieval Ireland*. Dublin: Columba, 2020.
58. Mc Gagh, Rosie. "Working in the Healing Industry with Fr Conlon," in *The Irish Catholic*. Dublin: Grace Communications Ltd (Feb. 27th 2020).
59. Macalister, Robert Alexander Stewart, ed. *Lebor Gabála Érenn: The Book of the Taking of Ireland*. Dublin: Irish Texts Society, 1932–1939.
60. Ó Corráin, Donnchadh, "Creating the Past: The Early Irish Genealogical Tradition." *Peritia*, vol. 12 (1998): 177–208.

61. Keating, Geoffrey. *The History of Ireland/Foras Feasa ar Éireann.* Translated by Edward Comyn and Patrick S. Dinneen. 1632: Ex-classics Project, 2009. http://www.exclassics.com.

62. Hughes, Felix J. "Eamhain Macha." *Seanchas Ardmhacha: Journal of the Armagh Diocesan Historical Society* 1, no. 2 (1955): 1–10.

63. Joyce, Patrick W., *A Smaller Social History of Ireland*, London: Longmans, Green, 1908.

64. Cameron, John. *The Gaelic Names for Plants.* Glasgow: John Mackay, 1900. Available online at https://wellcomecollection.org/works/x7k5kj6h/items

65. Kerr, James J., "Notes on Pharmacy in Old Dublin." *Dublin Historical Record*, vol. 4, (June–August 1942): 149–159.

66. FDA, Food & Drug Administration. *Biological Responses to Metal Implants.* A Collaborative Effort Amongst Subject Matter Experts (SMEs) Gathered from Across the Center for Devices and Radiological Health (CDRH), FDA, Maryland, September 2019. https://www.fda.gov › products-and-medical-procedures. Accessed 19th July 2020.

67. Sun, J., & Chen, W., "Music Therapy for Coma Patients: Preliminary Results." *European Review for Medical and Pharmacological Sciences*, vol. 19, no. 7 (2015): 1209–1218.

68. Leahy, Arthur Herbert. *Heroic Romances of Ireland, Translated into English Prose and Verse.* 1905, Available at https://www.sacred-texts.com/neu/hroi/hroiv1.htm

69. Rolleston, Thomas W., *Myths and Legends of the Celtic Race.* West Valley City, UT: Waking Lion Press. 2008.

70. Mac Firbisigh, Dubhaltach. *Leabhar mór na ngenealach: The great book of Irish genealogies*, compiled (1645–66) edited with translation and indexes by Nollaig Ó Muráile. Dublin: De Búrca, 2004.

71. Wycherly, Niamh. *The Cult of Relics in Early Medieval Ireland.* Turnhout, Belgium: Brepols, 2015.

72. Lucas, A. T. "The Social Role of Relics and Reliquaries in Ancient Ireland." *The Journal of the Royal Society of Antiquaries of Ireland* 116 (1986): 5–37.

73. Gesler, William. *Healing Places.* Maryland: Rowman & Littlefield, 2003.

74. Foley, Ronan. "Indigenous Narratives of Health: (Re)Placing Folk Medicine within Irish Health Histories." *Journal of Medical Humanities*, vol. 36, no. 1 (2015): 5–18.

75. Abram, David. "The Perceptual Implications of Gaia" *The Ecologist*, vol. 15, no. 3 (1985).

76. Ó Cadhla, Stiofáin. *The Holy Well Tradition. The Pattern of St. Declan, Ardmore, Co. Waterford, 1800–2000.* Maynooth: Four Courts Press, 2002.

77. Foley, Ronan. *Healing Waters: Therapeutic Landscapes in Historic and Contemporary Ireland.* Farnham: Ashgate. 2010.

78. Moerman, Daniel. *Meaning, Medicine and the Placebo Effect*, Cambridge: Cambridge University Press, 2002.

79. Thompson, Tok. "*Clocha Geala/Clocha Uaisle*: White Quartz in Irish Tradition" Béaloideas, vol. 73 (2005): 111–133.

80. Crawford, Ciara. "Disease and Illness in Medieval Ireland," PhD diss. NUI Maynooth, 2012.

81. MacArthur, William P., "The Identification of Some Pestilences Recorded in the Irish Annals." *Irish Historical Studies*, vol. 6, no. 23 (1949): 169–188.

82. Pierce A. Grace. "From Blefed to Scamach: Pestilence in Early Medieval Ireland." *Proceedings of the Royal Irish Academy: Archaeology, Culture, History, Literature* 118C (2018): 67–93.

83. Kelly, Maria. "'Unheard-of Mortality': The Black Death in Ireland." *History Ireland*, vol. 9, no. 4 (Winter 2001): 12–17.

84. Davies, Wendy. "The Place of Healing in Early Irish Society," in *Sages, Saints and Storytellers: Celtic studies in honour of Professor James Carney* Edited by D. ÓCorráin, L. Breatnach, and K. McCone, 43–55. Maynooth: An Sagart, 1989.

85. Beith, Mary. *Healing Threads. Traditional Medicines of the Highlands and Islands*. Edinburgh: Birlinn, 1995.

86. Shaw, Francis. "Medicine in Ireland in Medieval Times," in *What is Past is Prologue. A Retrospect of Irish Medicine*, Edited by W. Doolin and O. Fitzgerald. Dublin: Monument Press, 1952.

87. Kelly, F., *A Guide to Early Irish Law*. Dublin: Dublin Institute of Advanced Studies, 1988.

88. Binchy, Daniel A., "Lawyers and Chroniclers," in *Seven Centuries of Irish Learning*, Edited by B.Ó. Cúiv, Dublin: Thomas Davies Lectures, 1961.

89. Binchy, Daniel A., "Bretha Déin Chécht." *Ériu*, vol. 20 (1966): 1–66.

90. Dillon, Myles. *Celts and Aryans: Survivals of Indo-European Speech and Society*. Calcutta: Simla, Indian Institute of Advanced Study, 1975.

91. Dillon, Myles. "The Hindu Act of Truth in Celtic Tradition." *Modern Philogy*, vol. 44, no. 3 (1947): 137–140. Retrieved September 23, 2020, from http://www.jstor.org/stable/435296.

92. Dillon, Myles and Norah Chadwick, *The Celtic Realms*, London: Weidenfeld & Nicholson, 1967.

93. Kumar, Krishna, Kishan Singh, and Abhijit Patil, "The Clinical & Surgical Perspective of Tri-Marma." *European Journal of Pharmaceutical and Medical Research*, vol. 6, no. 5 (2019): 586–588.

94. Davergaon, Channamallikarjun. "Critical Review of Shankha Marma with Special Reference to the Pterion." *Journal of Ayurveda and Holistic Medicine*, vol. 5, no. 2 (2017): 24–28.

95. Kumari, Negi Vineeta, Parvat Susheela, Vyas Anju, Sharma Om. and Sharma S. K. *"Marma and Marma Therapy."* World Journal of Pharmaceutical Research, vol. 7, no. 15 (2018): 258–271.

96. Pal, Pradeep Kumar, Neera Saini, V. N. Mishra and H. H. Awasthi. "Critical Analysis of Lohitaksa Marma and its Applied Aspect." *European Journal of Pharmaceutical and Medical Research,* vol. 12 (2017): 350–353.

97. Verma, Jaydip Kumar. "Anatomical Consideration of Utkshepa Marma WSR to Ayurvedic and Modern Viewpoint." *International Ayurvedic Medical Journal,* vol. 6, no. 12 (December, 2018): 2344–2345.

98. Dalai, Sujit. "The Chapter "Marma Sharira" of Sushruta is Mirror of Surgery." *International Journal of Science & Healthcare Research,* vol. 4, issue 42 (2019): 62–69.

99. Ó Cuinn, Tadgh. *An Irish Book of Simple Medicines. Translated by Micheál* Ó Conchubhair. Dublin: School of Celtic Studies, Dublin Institute of Advance Studies, 1991.

100. Platearius, Mattheus. *The Livre des simples médecines (The book of simple medicines)* France 15th century. Facsimile with introduction and commentaries by, José María López Piñero, Natacha Elaguina, and Carlos Miranda. Barcelona: M. Moleiro, no date. Original in National library of Russia, St Petersburg.

101. Dundes, Alan. "The American Concept of Folklore." *Journal of the Folklore Institute,* vol. 3, no. 3 (special issue, The Yugoslav-AmericanFolklore Seminar) (Dec. 1966): 226–249.

102. Nic Dhonnchadha, Aoibheann. "The Medical School of Aghmacart, Queen's County." *Ossary, Laois and Leinster,* vol. 2 (2006): 11–43.

103. Dillon, Charlie. "Medical Practice in Gaelic Ireland," in *Ireland and Medicine in the Seventeeth and Eighteenth Centuries,* edited by J. Kelly and F. Clark, 39–52, Surrey: Ashgate, 2010.

104. Anderson, Frank J., *An Illustrated History of the Herbals.* Indiana: iUniverse, 1999.

105. Sheehan, Shaun. *An Irish Version of the Gaulterus de Dosibus.* Washington DC: Catholic University of America, 1938.

106. Nic Dhonnchadha, Aoibheann. "The 'Book of the O'Lees' and Other Medical Manuscripts and Astronomical Tracts," in *Treasures of the Royal Irish Academy Library,* Edited by B. Cunningham and S. Fitzpatrick, 81–92. Dublin: Royal Irish Academy, 2009.

107. Threlkeld, Caleb. *The First Irish Flora. Synopsis Stirpium Hibernicarum* Dublin: Davys, Norris & Worral 1726. Facsimile, Kilkenny: Boethius Press, 1988.

108. Wellcome, Henry S., *Medicine in Ancient Erin: An Historical Sketch from Celtic to Mediaeval Times.* London: Burroughs Wellcome, 1909.

109. Nelson, Charles. "Introduction," in *The First Irish Flora. Synopsis Stirpium Hibernicarum*. Kilkenny: Boethius Press 1988.

110. Williams, N., "A Note on John K'Eogh's 'Herbal'." *Eighteenth-Century Ireland/Iris an Dá Chultúr*, vol. 2 (1987): 198–202.

111. Harris, Jason, "Latin Learning and Irish Physicians, c1350–c1610," in *Rosa Anglica: Reassessments*, edited by Liam P. Ó Murchúhe, 1–25. London: Irish Texts Society, 2016.

112. Sõukand R, Mattalia G, Kolosova V, Stryamets N, Prakofjewa J, Belichenko O, Kuznetsova N, Minuzzi S, Keedus L, Prūse B, Simanova A, Ippolitova A, Kalle R. "Inventing a Herbal Tradition: The Complex Roots of the Current Popularity of *Epilobium Angustifolium* in Eastern Europe." *Journal of Ethnopharmacology*, vol. 247, (30th January, 2020): 112254.

113. Egan, F., "Irish Folk-Lore. Medical Plants." *The Folk-Lore Journal*, vol. 5, no. 1 (1887): 11–13.

114. Ó Muraíle, Nollaig. "The Hereditary Medical Families in Gaelic Ireland," in *Rosa Anglica: Reassessments*, edited by Liam P. Ó Murchú, 85–113. Irish Texts Society, Subsidiary Series 28, London: Irish Texts Society, 2016.

115. NFCS *0573: 005*. https://www.duchas.ie/en/cbes/4922268/4865880.

116. NFCS *0750: 105*. https://www.duchas.ie/en/cbes/5009136/4990098.

117. NFCS *0776C: 11_055*. https://www.duchas.ie/en/cbes/5260470/5256139.

118. Gerard, John. *The Herball, or General History of Plants*. London: J. Norton, 1597.

119. Mac Coitir, Niall. *Irish Wild Plants: Myths, Legends and Folklore*. Cork: Collins Press, 2006.

120. NFCS *0442: 468*. https://www.duchas.ie/en/cbes/4706337/4704062.

121. NFCS *157: 463*. https://www.duchas.ie/en/cbes/4701668/4691474.

122. Curtis, Patrick J., *The Lightning Tree*. Dingle: Brandon, 2008.

123. Ray, Celeste. "The Sacred and the Body Politic at Ireland's Holy Wells." *International Social Science Journal*, vol. 62, (2011): 205–206.

124. Abram, David. "The Perceptual Implications of Gaia." *The Ecologist*, vol. 15, no. 3 (1985): 96–103.

125. Briody, Mícheál. *The Irish Folklore Commission 1935–1970*. Helsinki: Finnish Literature Society, 2007.

126. NFC, *National Folklore Collection*. 1935 – present. https://www.duchas.ie.

127. NFCS *0746: 266*. https://www.duchas.ie/en/cbes/5009123/4988634.

128. NFCS *0931: 380*. https://www.duchas.ie/en/cbes/4758587/4756941.

129. NFCS *0199: 426*. https://www.duchas.ie/en/cbes/4602760/4602003.

130. NFCS *0252: 421*. https://www.duchas.ie/en/cbes/4798700/4791336.

131. NFCS *0802: 060*. https://www.duchas.ie/en/cbes/5044577/5023566.

132. NFCS *0752: 275*. https://www.duchas.ie/en/cbes/5009144/4991266.

133. NFCS *0803: 320*. https://www.duchas.ie/en/cbes/5044585/5024001.

134. NFCS *0532: 125*. https://www.duchas.ie/en/cbes/4922127/4854645.

135. Moses, Larry. "Legends by the Numbers: The Symbolism of Numbers in the 'Secret History of the Mongols.'" *Asian Folklore Studies,* vol. 55, no. 1, (1996): 73–97.

136. Moses, Larry. "Triplicated Triplets: The Number Nine in the 'Secret History' of the Mongols." *Asian Folklore Studies,* vol. 45, no. 2 (1986): 287–294.

137. NFCS *0534: 340*. https://www.duchas.ie/en/cbes/4922136/4855625.

138. NFCS *0270: 143*. https://www.duchas.ie/en/cbes/4811598/4800490.

139. NFCS *0270: 139*. https://www.duchas.ie/en/cbes/4811598/4800486.

140. NFCS *773: 048*. https://www.duchas.ie/en/cbes/4742157/4740788.

141. NFCS *0773: 048*. https://www.duchas.ie/en/cbes/4742157/4740788.

142. NFCS *0580: 155*. https://www.duchas.ie/en/cbes/4922300/4868255/5020135.

143. NFCS *0787: 52*. https://www.duchas.ie/en/cbes/4428183/4384598.

144. NFC *1838: 222; Informant:* Michael Rooney, Blacklion, Collector: P.J. Gaynor. Sept. 1974.

145. NFC *1838: 113; Informant:* Michael Rooney, Blacklion, Co. Cavan. Collector: P.J. Gaynor, September 1974.

146. Redman, Deborah, A., "Ruscus Aculeatus (Butcher's Broom) as a Potential Treatment for Orthostatic Hypotension, with a Case Report." *J Altern Complement Med.,* vol. 6, no. 6 (2000): 539–549.

147. NFCS *0592: 033*. https://www.duchas.ie/en/cbes/5177627/5174083/5199466.

148. NFCS *0661: 086*. https://www.duchas.ie/en/cbes/5008821/4958922.

149. NFCS *0768: 121*. https://www.duchas.ie/en/cbes/5009204/4997462/5104455.

150. NFCS *0877: 053*. https://www.duchas.ie/en/cbes/5009238/5000858/5122830.

151. NFCS *0150: 63*. https://www.duchas.ie/en/cbes/4428065/4374694/4461636.

152. NFC *1838: 161* Informant: James O'Reilly, Co. Louth. Collector: P.J. Gaynor. October 1974.

153. Roe, Helen, Maybury. "Tales, Customs and Belief from Laoighis." *Bealoideas,* 1939. vol. 9, no. 1 (June 1939): 21–35.

154. Lyons, William S., *Spirit Talkers: North American Indian Medicine Powers.* Kansas: Prayer Efficacy Publishing, 2012.

155. Eliade, Mircea. *Shamanism. Archaic Techniques of Ecstasy.* Princeton: Princeton University Press, 1964 (2004 edition).

156. NFC *744: 10;*

157. NFC *a54: 191*. Informant: J. Maher, Knockbyrne, Co. Wexford. Collector: T. O Ciardha. 21st March 1935.

158. Conlon, J Michael et al. "Potential Therapeutic Applications of Multifunctional Host-Defense Peptides from Frog Skin as Anti-Cancer, Anti-

Viral, Immunomodulatory, and Anti-Diabetic Agents." *Peptides*, vol. 57 (2014): 67–77.

159. Wing, Donna Marie. "A Comparison of Traditional Folk Healing Concepts with Contemporary Healing Concepts." *Journal of Community Health Nursing* vol. 15, no. 3 (1998): 143–54.

160. NFCS *0869: 228*. https://www.duchas.ie/en/cbes/4742039/4730129.

161. Moore, Ronnie. "A General Practice, A Country Practice: The Cure, the Charm and Informal Healing in Northern Ireland," in *Folk Healing and Health Care Practices in Britain and Ireland*, edited by R. Moore and S. McCLean, 104–129, Oxford: Berghahn Books, 2010.

162. Ó Giolláin, Diarmuid. "The Fairy Belief and Official Religion in Ireland," in *The Good People*, edited by P. Narváez, 199–214. Lexington: University Press of Kentucky, 1991.

163. Ó Súilleabháin, Seán. *Irish Folk Custom and Belief*. Dublin: Three Candles Ltd, 1967.

164. Glassie, Henry. *Passing the Time in Ballynemone*. Bloomington, Indiana: Indiana University Press, 1995.

165. Al-Sughayir, M.A., "*Public View of the "Evil Eye" and its Role in Psychiatry. A Study in Saudi Society*." The Arab Journal of Psychiatry, vol. 7 no. 2 (1996): 152–160.

166. Ó Súilleabháin, Seán. *Irish Folk Custom and Belief*. Dublin: Three Candles Press, 1967.

167. Goek, Sara. "From Ireland to the US: A Brief Migration History" *Irish Times*, Thurs. Oct. 29, 2015.

168. Ó Tuathaigh, Gearóid. *I mBéal an Bháis*. Cork: Cork University Press, 2015.

169. Lozada, Mariana, Ana Ladio, and Mariana Weigandt. "Cultural Transmission of Ethnobotanical Knowledge in a Rural Community of Northwestern Patagonia, Argentina." *Economic Botany*, vol. 60, no. 4 (Winter, 2006): 374–385.

170. Keaveny, Anna Maria. *Only the poor speak Irish*, (2011): Personal communication, Dublin.

171. Magan, Manchán. *Thirty-Two Words for Field*. Dublin: Gill, 2020.

172. Abram, David. *The Spell of the Sensuous. Perception and Language in a More-than-Human-World*. New York: Vintage Books, 1996.

173. McCarthy, Michael John Fitzgerald. *Priests and People in Ireland*. Dublin: Hodges & Figgis, 1902.

174. Larkin, Emmet. *The Historical Dimensions of Irish Catholicism*. New York: Arno Press, 1976.

175. Larkin, Emmet. "The Devotional Revolution in Ireland, 1850–75." *The American Historical Review*, vol. 77, no. 3 (1972): 625–652.

176. Hyde, Douglas. *The Necessity for De-Anglicising Ireland. Irish National Literary* Society, Dublin. November 25, 1892.

177. Ó Súilleabháin, Sean. *Irish Folk Custom and Belief.* Dublin: Three Candles, 1967.

178. Maloney, Micheal. *Irish Ethno-Botany and the Evolution of Medicine in Ireland.* Dublin: Gill & Son, 1919.

179. Quinlan, Christina. *Common Plants used in Medicine.* Dublin: Commissioners of National Education, 1919.

180. Foley, Tadg (Jude). *Medicinal and Perfumery Plants and Herbs in Ireland.* Dublin: M.H. Gill & Son, 1933.

181. O'Reilly, Joseph. "Essential Oils and Medicinal Herbs." *Studies,* An Irish Quarterly Review, vol. 22, no. 87 (September 1933): 373–388.

182. Eliade, Mircea. *Images and Symbols: Studies in Religious Symbolism.* New Jersey: Princeton University Press, 1991.

183. Li, Qing. "Effect of Forest Bathing Trips on Human Immune Function." *Environmental Health and Preventive Medicine,* vol. 15, no. 1 (2010): 9–17.

184. Light, Phyllis D., *Southern Folk Medicine.* Berkeley: North Atlantic Books, 2018.

185. Callan, Maeve B., "The Safest City of Refuge: Brigid the Bishop." in *Sacred Sisters Gender, Sanctity, and Power in Medieval Ireland,* 85–112. Amsterdam: Amsterdam University Press, 2020.

186. Patterson, T.G.F., "Brigid's Crosses in County Armagh." *Ulster Journal of Archeology,* vol. 8 (1945): 43–8.

187. Danaher, Kevin. *The Year in Ireland.* Cork: The Mercier Press, 1972.

188. St. Clair, Sheila. *Folklore of the Ulster People.* 1971, Cork: Mercier Press, 1971.

189. Eliade, Mircea. *Patterns in Comparative Religion (Trans. R. Sheed).* London: Sheed & Ward, 1958.

190. NFCS *447: 192.* https://www.duchas.ie/en/cbes/4706356/4705793.

191. Swift, Jonathen. *The Journal to Stella,* edited by G.A. Aitken, London: Methuen, 1713.

192. Croker, Thomas C., *The Popular Songs of Ireland.* London: Henry Colburn, 1839.

193. NFCS *0004: 26.* https://www.duchas.ie/en/cbes/4602676/4594517.

194. Little, Kitty. *Kitty Little's Book of Herbal Beauty.* London: Penguin, 1981.

195. Boate, Gerard. *The Natural History of Ireland.* 1726. Available at https://celt.ucc.ie//published/E650002–001/.

196. NFCS *0527: 046.* https://www.duchas.ie/en/cbes/4922108/4852794.

197. NFCS *0846: 326.* https://www.duchas.ie/en/cbes/4758505/4749551.

198. NFCS *003: 192.* https://www.duchas.ie/en/cbes/4602675/4594475.

199. NFCS *0781: 108.* https://www.duchas.ie/en/cbes/4769975/4763587.

200. NFCS *0690: 118*. https://www.duchas.ie/en/cbes/5008928/4967235.
201. NFCS *0413: 205*. https://www.duchas.ie/en/cbes/4666602/4665830.
202. MacNeill, Máire. *The Festival of Lughnasa*. Dublin: Comhairle Bhéaloideas Éireann, 2008.
203. NFCS *0883: 114*. https://www.duchas.ie/en/cbes/5009267/5003092.
204. NFCS *0739: 234*. https://www.duchas.ie/en/cbes/5009095/4985966.
205. NFCS *0527: 042*. https://www.duchas.ie/en/cbes/4922108/4852790.
206. Mouhid, Lamia et al. "Yarrow Supercritical Extract Exerts Antitumoral Properties by Targeting Lipid Metabolism in Pancreatic Cancer." *PloS one*, vol. 14, no. 3 (March 26, 2019): e0214294.
207. Kenner, Dan and Yves Requena. *Botanical Medicine. A European Professional Perspective*. Massachusetts: Paradigm Publications, 1996.
208. Andrzej Sidor and Anna Gramza Michalowska. "Advanced research on the antioxidant and health benefit of elderberry (*Sambucus nigra*) in food—a review." *Journal of Functional Foods*, vol. 18, part B (2015): 941–958.
209. NFCS *1026: 032*. https://www.duchas.ie/en/cbes/4428247/4388248.
210. NFCS *0143: 531*. https://www.duchas.ie/en/cbes/4428039/4371242.
211. NFCS *0221: 644*. https://www.duchas.ie/en/cbes/4658432/4655079.
212. NFCS *0230: 195*. https://www.duchas.ie/en/cbes/4758451/4745084.
213. NFCS *0232: 097*. https://www.duchas.ie/en/cbes/4798653/4787203/4818751.
214. NFCS *0847: 529*. https://www.duchas.ie/en/cbes/4758508/4750155.
215. NFCS *0858: 094*. https://www.duchas.ie/en/cbes/4758549/4753873.
216. NFCS *0858: 101*. https://www.duchas.ie/en/cbes/4758549/4753880.
217. NFCS *0850: 118*. https://www.duchas.ie/en/cbes/4758519/4751018.
218. NFCS *0764: 436*. https://www.duchas.ie/en/cbes/5009188/4995906.
219. NFCS *0650: 276*. https://www.duchas.ie/en/cbes/4428148/4381915.
220. NFCS *0165: 158*. https://www.duchas.ie/en/cbes/4701695/4693415.
221. Adav, Kulveer Singhy, and Bijendra Kumer Singh, "Marigold : A Crop Having Great Medicinal Importance." *Advances in Life Sciences*, vol. 6, no. 1 (2017):
222. Mohammad, Sharrif Moghaddasi and Hamed Haddad Kashanisup. "Pot Marigold (*Calendula officinalis*) Medicinal Usage and Cultivation." *Scientific Research and Essays*, vol. 7, no. 14 (2012): 1468–72.
223. NFCS *0897: 154*. https://www.duchas.ie/en/cbes/5009325/5007225.
224. NFCS *0792: 444*. https://www.duchas.ie/en/cbes/4498840/4385948.
225. NFCS *0527: 044*. https://www.duchas.ie/en/cbes/4922108/4852792.
226. NFCS *0057: 0123*. https://www.duchas.ie/en/cbes/4583339/4580956.
227. NFCS *0764: 436*. https://www.duchas.ie/en/cbes/5009188/4995906.
228. NFCS *233: 095*. https://www.duchas.ie/en/cbes/5162102/5154217.

229. Zhang, Yukun, et al., "Modulatory Effect of Althaea Officinalis L Root Extract on Cisplatin-Induced Cytotoxicity and Cell Proliferation in A549 Human Lung Cancer Cell Line." *Tropical Journal of Pharmaceutical Research*, vol. 15, no. 12 (2016): 2647–2652.

230. NFCS *0013: 091*. https://www.duchas.ie/en/cbes/4591091/4589767/4615410.

231. NFCS *0979: 199*. https://www.duchas.ie/en/cbes/5044843/5043595.

232. NFCS *0710: 145*. https://www.duchas.ie/en/cbes/5008991/4974815/5112925.

233. NFCS *0349: 224*. https://www.duchas.ie/en/cbes/4921724/4893907/5183609.

234. NFCS *0639: 25*. https://www.duchas.ie/en/cbes/5277706/5276725/5277807.

235. NFCS *0794: 223*. https://www.duchas.ie/en/cbes/4428214/4386479/4456492.

236. NFCS *0853: 341*. https://www.duchas.ie/en/cbes/4758529/4752194/4782655.

237. NFCS *0107: 392*. https://www.duchas.ie/en/cbes/4427887/4354515/4551465.

238. NFCS *0214: 045*. https://www.duchas.ie/en/cbes/4649701/4648566/4652200.

239. NFCS *0013: 255*. https://www.duchas.ie/en/cbes/4591092/4589931/4623920.

240. NFCS *0587: 191*. https://www.duchas.ie/en/cbes/5177608/5172983.

241. Staiger, Christiane. "Comfrey: a Clinical Overview." *Phytotherapy Research: PTR*, vol. 26, no. 10 (2012): 1441–8.

242. NFCS *1000: 098*. https://www.duchas.ie/en/cbes/5070789/5063631.

243. NFCS *0159:289*. https://www.duchas.ie/en/cbes/4701677/4692026/4726621.

244. NFCS *0849: 351*. https://www.duchas.ie/en/cbes/4758517/4750870/4955454.

245. NFCS *0657: 248*. https://www.duchas.ie/en/cbes/5008805/4957738/5070947.

246. NFCS *0706: 069*. https://www.duchas.ie/en/cbes/5008980/4973304/5111308.

247. NFCS *289: 313*. https://www.duchas.ie/en/cbes/4921600/4883509/5149408.

248. Chan, Yuk-Shing et al. "A review of the pharmacological effects of *Arctium lappa* (burdock)." *Inflammopharmacology*, vol. 19, no. 5 (2011): 245–54.

249. NFCS *0858: 094*. https://www.duchas.ie/en/cbes/4758549/4753873.

250. NFCS *0480: 375.* https://www.duchas.ie/en/cbes/4921935/4911358/4932681.
251. NFCS *0142: 303.* https://www.duchas.ie/en/cbes/4476321/4370747/4476387.
252. NFCS *0883:182.* https://www.duchas.ie/en/cbes/5009269/5003161/5131805.
253. NFCS *0650:143.* https://www.duchas.ie/en/cbes/4428146/4381737.
254. NFCS *0115: 281.* https://www.duchas.ie/en/cbes/4427922/4357817/4454054.
255. NFCS *0853: 321.* https://www.duchas.ie/en/cbes/4758529/4752174/4782655.
256. Wirngo, Fonyuy E. et al. "The Physiological Effects of Dandelion (*Taraxacum Officinale*) in Type 2 Diabetes." *The review of diabetic studies: RDS*, vol. 13, no. 2–3 (2016): 113–131.
257. NFCS, *0155: 283.* https://www.duchas.ie/en/cbes/4701656/4690539/4707167.
258. Sigstedt, Sophia C et al. "Evaluation of Aqueous Extracts of Taraxacum Officinale on Growth and Invasion of Breast and Prostate Cancer Cells." *International Journal of Oncology,* vol. 32, no. 5 (May, 2008): 1085–90.
259. Ross, Jonathan. *A Clinical Materia Medica.* 2010, Germany: Verlag fur Ganzheitliche Medizin Dr. Erich Wuhr GmbH.
260. NFCS *0454: 012.* https://www.duchas.ie/en/cbes/4713243/4710924/4726702.
261. NFCS *0948: 006.* https://www.duchas.ie/en/cbes/4723858/4719648/4760405.
262. NFCS *736: 022.* https://www.duchas.ie/en/cbes/5009080/4984590.
263. Malinowski B, Zalewska K, Węsierska A, et al. "Intermittent Fasting in Cardiovascular Disorders, An Overview." *Nutrients,* vol. 11, no. 3 (2019): 673.
264. Moore, Ronnie and Stuart McLean, eds. *Folk Healing and Health Care Practices in Britain and Ireland.* New York: Berghahn Books, 2010.

INDEX